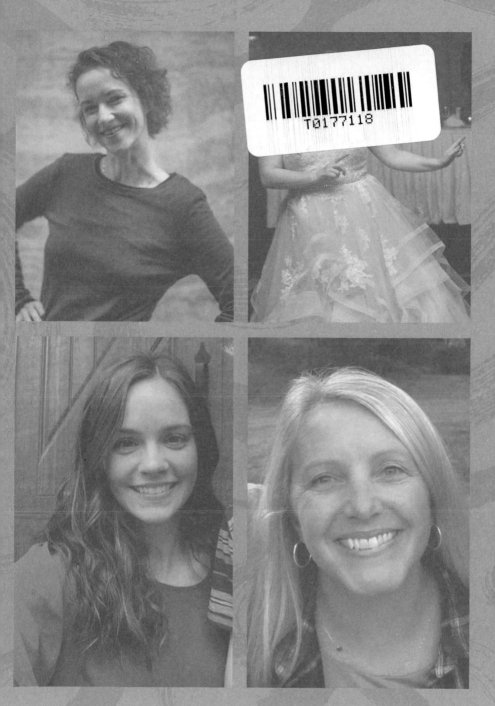

RIE ANAMI | NATASHA LAM | EMILY HOFFMAN
CATHERINE GREEN | TARA CASSAGRANDE | KADIANA VEGEE
CASSIE WALKER | CHRISTINA BRUCE-BENNION

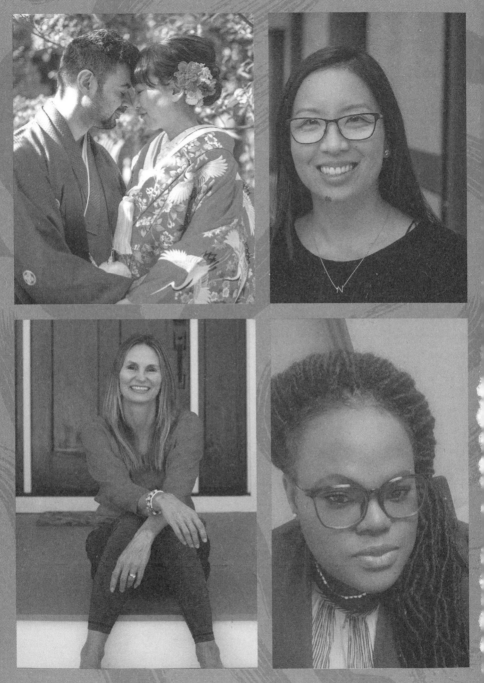

Several survivors offered stories in addition to those individuals named in the book. Your wisdom and words created content and context and I cannot thank you enough for your courage and vulnerability.

ENOUGH

Cervical cancer kills almost 350,000 women each year. What's more horrifying is that millions have died of a disease that's nearly 100 percent preventable. It's no secret that health care is full of inequities, with a severe lack of accessible screening programs. But women's health care is also impeded by cultural, gender, and political barriers, issues that have combined to create devastating consequences.

A leading expert in cervical cancer prevention, Dr. Linda Eckert takes her years of experience and weaves them together with the voices of the courageous women who use their own experience of cervical cancer to advocate for change. This heartbreaking, yet hopeful, book takes you through the world of cervical cancer with evidence-based information, personal stories, and actionable outcomes. Society flourishes when women have access to safe and affordable health care. Together we can make this need a reality and eliminate the world's most preventable cancer.

Dr. Linda Eckert is a Professor of Obstetrics and Gynecology with an Infectious Disease Fellowship at the University of Washington and an internationally recognized expert in immunizations and cervical cancer prevention. For over thirty years, Dr. Eckert has worked at Seattle's Harborview hospital, treating people from all around the world. Frequently in the spotlight for her expertise in HPV vaccinations and cervical cancer screenings, Dr. Eckert is passionate in her drive to eliminate this deadly disease.

"Beautifully written, Enough *is a searing call to arms, for too many women are dying of cervical cancer when we have the tools to save their lives. The unnecessary human cost of cervical cancer is a scandal, and one that Dr. Eckert is determined to fix."*

Nicholas Kristof, Columnist,
New York Times and co-author, *Half the Sky*

"Eckert presents an urgent and powerful call to action to save lives, based on her decades of practice and research around the world. Enough *is an essential resource for anyone concerned with public health, women's rights, and addressing racial and national inequities in health care."*

Anjli Parrin, Director, Global Human Rights Clinic,
University of Chicago Law School

"This is a beautifully written, powerful tale of truth and hope, as Dr. Eckert combines her authoritative work with cervical cancer prevention alongside the inspiring voices of women from all over the world."

Princess Nono Simelela, former
WHO Assistant Director General for Strategic Priorities

"Cervical cancer cannot be a disease of inequities anymore and the role of this book is crucial to always remember this. Thanks to the author for this essential piece of advocacy."

Dr. Nathalie Broutet, MD, PhD, Lead of the Cervical
Cancer Elimination Initiative (2005–2022),
WHO Department of Sexual and Reproductive Health and Rights

"A book to read, to gift, to pass on to friends and those who need to know, to USE to make change–Dr. Eckert deftly intertwines the barriers to achieving [cervical cancer elimination], the science and financial issues as well as cultural issues and the bewildering continuing disvaluing of women's rights and lives."

Joanna M. Cain, MD, Professor (retired) University of Massachusetts
and Co Chair, Cervical Cancer subcommittee International
Federation of Gynecology and Obstetrics (FIGO)

"Dr. Eckert details moving and powerful stories of women battling cervical cancer. Many will bring you to tears, especially as Dr. Eckert educates us that nearly all of the cancers are preventable. In the end she gives us a hopeful roadmap to address health inequities and systems challenges that would allow us to end this deadly cancer."

Barbara Goff, MD, Professor and Chair, Department of Obstetrics and Gynecology, UW Medicine, Surgeon-in-Chief, University of Washington Medical Center

"Cervical cancer is a preventable disease. Enough *is the book that should be put in the hands of anyone who has received a [cervical cancer] diagnosis or is supporting someone with a diagnosis."*

Diana Rivington, emeritus of the Canadian International Development Agency (CIDA)

"As those with cervical cancer tell their stories, cervical cancer becomes real. This story could be your sister, your mother, your daughter, your aunt, your life partner. Cervical cancer strikes in Zambia, or in Canada, in Honduras, or Australia. In Enough *these individuals, whose stories are wonderfully expressed, come to life."*

Karen Nakawala, cervical cancer survivor, Founder of Teal Sisters, Zambia

"I would strongly recommend this book to anyone seeking to learn more about cervical cancer, especially those developing health policies."

Dr. Aisha Jumaan, Founder and President of Yemen Relief and Reconstruction Foundation, Previous director of the HPV Vaccines: Evidence of Impact project

"This book opened my eyes so wide and showed the whole world what cervical cancer is. All aspects, all successes, all failures."

Icó Tóth, President, Mallow Flower Foundation, Hungary

"Intimate, and informative, Enough *reminds us that the choice to end cervical cancer belongs to each of us. Now is the time to act."*

Heather White, Executive Director, TogetHER for Health, www.togetherforhealth.org

"This book serves as a powerful resource to educate medical professionals and the public alike to take charge of self-care and work toward a cervical cancer-free world."

Dr. Shobha S. Krishnan, Founder and President, Global Initiative Against HPV and Cervical Cancer

Enough

Because We Can Stop Cervical Cancer

DR. LINDA ECKERT

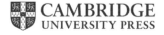

CAMBRIDGE
UNIVERSITY PRESS

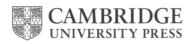

Shaftesbury Road, Cambridge CB2 8EA, United Kingdom

One Liberty Plaza, 20th Floor, New York, NY 10006, USA

477 Williamstown Road, Port Melbourne, VIC 3207, Australia

314–321, 3rd Floor, Plot 3, Splendor Forum, Jasola District Centre, New Delhi – 110025, India

103 Penang Road, #05–06/07, Visioncrest Commercial, Singapore 238467

Cambridge University Press is part of Cambridge University Press & Assessment, a department of the University of Cambridge.

We share the University's mission to contribute to society through the pursuit of education, learning and research at the highest international levels of excellence.

www.cambridge.org
Information on this title: www.cambridge.org/9781009412650

DOI: 10.1017/9781009412681

First published 2024

Printed in Mexico by Litográfica Ingramex, S.A. de C.V.

A catalogue record for this publication is available from the British Library

A Cataloging-in-Publication data record for this book is available from the Library of Congress

ISBN 978-1-009-41265-0 Hardback

Additional resources for this publication at www.cambridge.org/xxx

Cambridge University Press & Assessment has no responsibility for the persistence or accuracy of URLs for external or third-party internet websites referred to in this publication and does not guarantee that any content on such websites is, or will remain, accurate or appropriate.

Every effort has beenmade in preparing this book to provide accurate and up-to-date information that is in accord with accepted standards and practice at the time of publication. Although case histories are drawn from actual cases, the author has changed names of some patients and altered potentially identifying details about them. The author has also reconstructed scenes and created composite stories from thirty years of patient care experiences. Nevertheless, the authors, editors, and publishers canmake nowarranties that the information contained herein is totally free from error, not least because clinical standards are constantly changing through research and regulation. The authors and publishers therefore disclaim all liability for direct or consequential damages resulting from the use of material contained in this book. Readers are strongly advised to pay careful attention to information provided by the manufacturer of any drugs or equipment that they plan to use.

I dedicate this book to my patients, and to the survivors who shared their stories. By welcoming me into your lives – you have changed mine.

May your words change the futures of many.

CONTENTS

FIGURES

THE CALLING

I was working as a doctor in a makeshift Nicaraguan clinic. My physician-husband and I were part of a volunteer medical group offering short-term care to rural residents. Under a roofed veranda that wrapped around a local school, we'd set up services roughly three hours by car from the nearest large town. A small breeze flowed between the veranda's pillars, offering faint relief from the heat.

Each of our group of five – two physicians and three nurse-practitioners – had a small table and two chairs, along with basic medical equipment, such as blood pressure cuffs and stethoscopes. We sat with our backs to the privacy screens we'd roughly constructed using long curtains suspended from rods surrounding and separating two examination tables intended only for the sickest of patients. Because our clinic only offered primary care screening and basic medications like Tylenol or treatment for high blood pressure, we lacked rudimentary equipment for pelvic examinations, let alone the ability to conduct specialized exams on women exhibiting signs of cervical cancer.

My husband and I spoke with patients, one by one. Some had come to exercise a rare opportunity to ask a doctor or nurse a question or obtain long-awaited medication. Most appeared energetic and well. They chatted eagerly with neighbors and friends while waiting in a long line snaking out of sight beyond the edge of the school.

As I was soon to find out, others had made the long trip – many on foot – because they had far more pressing concerns. They'd found a way to get there, even if that meant using innovative forms of transport for ailing family members. Several mothers, for instance, carted children in wheelbarrows padded with blankets. I had not witnessed any strollers in this rural area, imagining the difficulties of navigating a stroller through rutted dirt roads.

As word got through the crowd that I was an obstetrician and gynecologist, my queue shifted predominantly to female patients. Many came with questions about painful periods, contraception, or how to improve their chances for pregnancy.

How I First Met Maria

We had been attending to patients for several hours when I noticed a commotion in my patient line. From near the back, a middle-aged man was pushing a wheelbarrow cart with a grown woman folded into it. She barely fit, the wheelbarrow too small to hold an adult body, her legs dangling over the side, her feet sometimes bumping the ground. The man worked steadily to move the two of them up through that long line. His brow was furrowed, and he was sweating from the effort. I watched him ask over and over if he could move the two of them up to the front. When he arrived, I could see that the woman looked dangerously pale and thin.

"Her name is Maria," the man said. "She is my wife." I got out of my chair and moved toward them, and together we wheeled Maria back to one of the examination tables. "I'm very worried about her," Maria's husband told me. "She is losing weight and has little energy to take care of our three children." When we moved Maria to the table, I noticed a dark, circular stain on the back of her skirt. She had been sitting on a rag stained the same purplish-black color. The rag and skirt stains looked and smelled like old blood.

I asked Maria about her medical history. She was forty years old, although I would have guessed fifty. She'd been having back pain and abnormal vaginal discharge for months. The last three or four months, the discharge had become bloodier and a bright red color some days, darker other days. Unlike the flow from her period, this bloody discharge was constant. She'd had no trouble with her urine or bowel movements but was feeling exhausted all the time.

I finally asked the question I'd been dreading because I felt I knew the answer: "Maria, have you ever had an examination called a Pap smear? Or any type of examination of your vagina or opening to your womb?" She and her husband looked at me blankly.

"We had midwives for our babies," her husband said proudly. I would learn that Maria's experience was typical of many women in lower-income countries, who only get medical care when they're pregnant – if then.

"I would like to do a gentle examination of your vagina with my fingers," I told Maria. "To see if I can learn anything about your bleeding." I covered Maria's waist and legs using a sheet from the exam table. I helped her gently slide down her undergarments, had her open her legs with her knees falling apart, and, using the two gloved fingers of my right hand underneath the sheet, I slowly examined her vagina. At the top, smooth tissue gave way to a firm and irregularly bordered mass five centimeters across and extending outside her cervix and into the vaginal tissue.

My heart sank. I was sure Maria had cervical cancer.

The Stark Realities for Lower-Income Countries

In this isolated area, I lacked the means and equipment to offer Maria anything more. The nearest regional hospital could confirm the presence of cervical cancer with a biopsy, but even a reliable diagnosis provided no guarantee the hospital had the means to treat her cancer.

What should I tell Maria and her husband? How could I help? I told them I was worried something was growing at the top of Maria's vagina that should not be there and urged her to see the specialist in town. I asked her husband if he knew anyone who could give them a ride to the central hospital.

As her husband stepped out from the curtained area to ask for a ride, Maria turned to me. "Doctor, tell me, do I have cancer?"

I took a deep breath. "I cannot know for sure without doing a biopsy," I told her. "That is why I want you to get further testing and treatment. But I am very worried."

With an audible groan, she closed her eyes and turned her head away from me. I could feel her chest moving with quiet sobs as my hand rested on her shoulder. We stayed there, silent, for what seemed like several minutes. Maria took a breath, rolled her head back to look at me, and through both of our tears we held each other's gaze in mute understanding.

Then Maria breathed in again, her lips pursed, and with a grunt she tried to push herself up on her elbows. She seemed to be summoning resolve to face her prognosis. Too weak to sit up on her own, she asked for help getting dressed. I guided her back into her wheelbarrow. By then, her husband had come back, saying he'd found a ride into town for the two of them.

He pushed her back out into the crowd, and I watched the back of Maria's head rise and fall with the ruts in the road. I never saw Maria again.

Cervical Cancer Ruthless – but Preventable

It was the fall of 1991 when I met Maria, but I cannot forget her. I can close my eyes and capture the image of her rolling away in that unpainted wooden wheelbarrow, her feet bumping against the rutted road. I can retreat to my core and feel my hand on her shoulder, Maria quaking with quiet sobs as she came to grasp her diagnosis. I vividly remember the moment of profound connection when our eyes met, and without words, she told me she knew about the progression of her disease, that it would soon rob her of her future.

I wish I could say that meeting Maria was a one-time experience, but it's not. Working and traveling worldwide throughout my decades of caring for women as an obstetrician and gynecologist, I have seen too many *Marias* – women with advanced cervical cancer in a setting where treatment is either sparse, too expensive, or unavailable altogether, as it was in rural Nicaragua in 1991.

But I have encountered other *Marias* in all settings, across oceans, above and below the equator, in clinics where women came dressed in expensive designer shoes, and in dusty village squares where patients wore plastic flip-flops. I have met *Marias* in Texas, where I received my residency training and then worked in a farm workers' clinic on the Rio Grande border. Some *Marias* I met while working in Africa - both caring for patients and as a consultant helping African health departments design their cervical cancer prevention programs. Other *Marias* I have encountered in Seattle, where I've had the privilege of providing care for over thirty years in a women's clinic at Harborview, the largest public hospital in the Pacific Northwest. Sadly, I can say that *Maria* lives in all places, all settings, and has been present with me my entire professional life.

And while the *Marias* have left an indelible mark on my spirit and heart, by contrast, I want to lose sight of their killer, cervical cancer - a demon I would dearly love for this world to exorcize. I am keenly aware that this task is too big for one person. The onward march of cervical cancer - its deft thievery of lives, the vitality it steals from its victims, their families, their communities, from all of us - shows no sign of abating. Despite any efforts to stop it, cervical cancer is relentless and ever-increasing.

And yet, this form of cancer *should* leave. This relentless cancer that strikes women in the prime of their lives, this stealth killer that is especially skilled at striking the unsuspecting individual who may have never heard of it, or did not know it could be prevented, or did not have access to the health care that could prevent it - this cancer *should* leave.

Be gone, cervical cancer. Release your death grip on women.
You are a preventable cancer, after all.

Stop for a minute. Take that in: "a preventable cancer." Just think how rare it is to have those two words, *preventable* and *cancer*, together in one phrase. What does that mean?

Well, it means that medical providers know what causes cervical cancer, how to treat it and cure it if it's found early enough, and how to prevent it. Cervical cancer is a cancer that could be eliminated, that need not exist at all. Yet, this preventable cancer kills a woman somewhere in the world every two minutes. That translates to 360 women dying a day.

Women dying. From a preventable cancer. Three hundred and forty thousand deaths a year. Six hundred thousand persons with cervixes diagnosed a year – and, if they do not die of cervical cancer, the treatment leaves permanent scars on both body and soul.

My Journey toward "Enough"

I've finally reached a place in my personal and professional life where I can no longer stand by and witness so much suffering. I need to shout out to the world from the rooftops: *Enough! Enough Marias. Enough unnecessary death and suffering.*

I can no longer tolerate hundreds of needless deaths a day, because my career has allowed me to follow the near-miraculous advancements of cervical cancer prevention. As a consultant for the World Health Organization for more than a decade and one of the recent authors of a set of global recommendations aimed at eliminating cervical cancer, I know it's possible to offer increasingly effective screening tests for this disease, both to lower-income countries and to impoverished, marginalized communities in higher-income countries. I know that these tests can pick up pre-cancerous abnormalities in persons with cervixes, and that effective treatments can resolve pre-cancer before it becomes cancer. I know that these treatments, just as with screening, can work within communities and countries of all financial and medical means. I know that if a person has developed cervical cancer and it's found early enough, the cure rate is excellent. And perhaps even more astonishing, I know we already have a terrific, lifesaving vaccine that can prevent more than 90 percent of cervical cancer. And yet, with innumerable ways to prevent these 360 deaths a day, we continue to let them happen.

Enough, I think to myself. *Surely – surely if people just heard the stories of the amazing women I've met, the patients I've cared for, they, too, would be moved.* In publishing this book, I thought I could open people's eyes once they'd heard from the brave women who stepped forward and allowed me to tell their cervical cancer stories – that sharing their suffering might prevent further suffering, further death.

I write these words and share other women's stories with humility, knowing that as I've tried to convey the voices and perspectives of many people – patients, clinic providers, community leaders, journalists, professors, and politicians – I also have my own personal perspective and beliefs to share. I write with the hope of finding like-minded others, no matter their background, country of origin, or personal circumstances.

I am a woman raised in the western United States, in a country where I had the opportunity to go to college and medical school and pursue advanced medical training. I am White, and I am talking about a disease that kills more women of color. In addition to working in medical clinics in my own country, labeled "high-income" by the World Bank, I have lived and worked as a physician in Liberia, Nicaragua, and Kenya – countries deemed "low-income." While I am a passionate advocate for those who have been attacked by this cancer, I am not a cervical cancer survivor. I've never had to fight to obtain health care. I am acutely aware that my perspective arises, in part, from a place of privilege.

I own my perspective as a physician who has provided patient care to women for decades across many countries and within communities filled with women of varying needs and financial means. Caring for women and bearing witness to their courage as they confront illness; witnessing their immense power as they birth children; being privy to their deepest concerns in moments of profound vulnerability: my role in these women's lives has been, and continues to be, my deepest privilege and my greatest inspiration. I am a fierce believer in the power of women.

I also own my perspective as a person whose cervical cancer expertise reflects my work with thousands of female patients, in conducting research on infectious diseases in women, and, by assisting the WHO to develop policies that improve access to and understanding of the human papillomavirus (HPV) vaccines (Box I.1), a critical tool in cervical cancer prevention, and cervical cancer prevention guidelines to enable countries to lower their death rates from cervical cancer. I have worked in consultation with the health ministries of several African countries, such as Namibia, Malawi, and Botswana, toward developing their own cervical cancer prevention guidelines. This work has offered me a place at the table with global leaders and researchers focused on preventing cervical cancer worldwide and has allowed me to have everyday conversations and interactions with those who oversee important cervical cancer screening in African clinics located in Namibia or in Malawi.

While I have written many academic articles and textbook chapters, presented data at international meetings, given countless lectures, and taught budding doctors and medical students how to do pelvic examinations and deliver babies, I have never

---

Box I.1

HPV vaccines bolster the immune system to offer protection against HPV infections. Because HPV is sexually transmitted, the vaccine offers maximum protection against the types of HPV infection that can cause cervical cancer when it is given before initial exposure to HPV – essentially when persons with cervixes are young or before they've had sex for the first time. The vaccine also creates a stronger immune response in girls under fifteen and requires fewer vaccine doses. That's why the World Health Organization recommends giving the HPV vaccine to nine- to fourteen-year-old girls.

written a book like this, geared toward a non-medical audience, about a disease that should not exist but continues to kill.

But I must do my part, knowing it will take a far-reaching, global effort to conquer this cancer. I'm willing to spread the word to anyone who will hear it. That word, the word that pushes me to keep going, is the title of this book: *Enough.*

Enough, because cervical cancer can be stopped.
Enough, because each of us can play a role in making it stop.

And, because my former patient, Maria, isn't here to say this out loud, I will speak on her behalf by saying that women are worth it. All women are worth the effort. Intrinsically, we all know that. But it will take all of us – working together – to show how passionately we believe it.

Part One
A Preventable Cancer

1 THE POTENT PROMISE AND THE ROTTEN REALITY

She was my last patient of a busy morning. Her morning call to our clinic – "my bleeding just won't quit" – earned her the 11:40 a.m. slot, held open for patients with urgent matters. Her name was Susie.

As I would later learn, Susie was forty-six years old but hadn't seen a nurse or doctor for seven years. She'd moved around from state to state a few times, been briefly employed in the service industry, but never stayed in one place long enough or earned enough to qualify for ongoing medical care. The last place she'd gone for care, a community health clinic in Colorado, had offered subsidized care, but funding issues had forced it to close.

Like many women, Susie never put Pap smear appointments high on her list. "I should go get a check-up," she'd thought to herself. But such *shoulds* are rarely enough for patients like Susie to overcome daunting obstacles, including expensive medical fees, difficulty finding a clinic reasonably close to home, and perhaps most of all, the ability to trust a doctor with such an intimate procedure. Susie had been sexually assaulted. Women already feel vulnerable sitting on an exam table covered only by a sheet, knees spread apart for an internal pelvic examination – such vulnerability can be unimaginable for a woman who has experienced sexual violence.

Ideally, medical clinics offer patients a sense of safety, lessening their ambivalence about important exams. Our examination rooms in this clinic were small, equivalent to the interiors of Volkswagen vans. They held four-drawer, waist-high storage

cabinets whose compartments hid pieces of equipment that
could make women anxious, especially the metal speculums.
Shaped like a duck's bill, a speculum enables examiners to
gently hold the vaginal walls in place for viewing the cervix –
the vaginal opening to the uterus. The examination tables in our
clinic were positioned to offer privacy, with the foot of the table
farthest from the door. Fuzzy, colorful footies covering the
stirrups where clients rested their feet provided extra padding
and a sense of comfort.

Unfortunately, none of these factors made much difference
in bringing Susie to our clinic – a woman from out of town, who,
for a variety of reasons beyond her control, had waited too long
to take advantage of the clinic's preventative cancer care. It
didn't help that on that busy clinic day I'd had less opportunity
to prepare for a patient like Susie. I'd only had time to read my
medical assistant's brief note, telling me that Susie had had "no
medical care for seven years," "irregular vaginal bleeding for
three months," and a "swollen right leg for six weeks."

As I stood outside the exam room where Susie was waiting,
my assistant approached me. "I did not want to write this on the
chart," she whispered, "but the room really smells." I waited for
more. "Susie told me she's scared something is really wrong."

When something is wrong, the patient is often the first to
know.

The Moment Medical Training Rarely Prepares You For

As I cracked open the door to the exam room, the odor rushed
out and overtook me. It was the smell of rottenness, the pungent smell of tissue dying. I knew that smell. As I listened to
Susie's story, I sensed the diagnosis even before doing the exam:
cervical cancer.

The odor was not lost on Susie. She sat in a chair beside the
exam table, her face red, her eyes toward the floor. It occurred to
me that her shame was probably one reason she'd waited so long

to go to a doctor, hoping her condition would improve before she had to have an embarrassing, traumatic examination, her vagina smelling of rottenness. But her condition did not improve. She told me she'd thought the smell came from bleeding for so long.

I asked Susie to tell me more about her leg swelling. *Only swollen on the right. Gradually getting worse. No, no calf pain* that might go with a blood clot but a generalized ache, *especially at the end of the day. Maybe some back pain, worse, also, on the right side of the back.*

As I listened, I carefully considered how to do this examination in the least distressing way. I was 99 percent sure I'd find a mass at the top of her vagina and that I'd want to take a biopsy to confirm what my heart and gut were so sure of already. Since Susie had been bleeding for so long, I'd also need to prepare for increased bleeding with the biopsy. Should the bleeding become heavy, I'd need to ask for help.

By now, Susie's morning appointment had wound into early afternoon. I told her I'd need consent for the biopsies. Susie's back stiffened, and she leaned forward in her chair. Her lips tightened, and I could see her brow knitting. As I got up to leave, I felt her anxiety. It had a presence, hanging thick in the air, mixing with the pungent odor.

Our clinic was on lunch hour, so I gathered up the necessary equipment by myself, and peeked into our medical provider room. My colleague, Samantha, was sitting there typing away. "Sammie, I'm about to do a biopsy on a woman, and I'm afraid she could bleed a lot. Can you please come in the room with me?" Sammie rose with a quick nod. As she opened the door to the room where Susie waited, we were again greeted by the odor. *That odor.* Sammie turned back to me with empathy and a knowing look in her eyes.

I introduced Sammie to Susie. While Susie lay on the exam table and I positioned her in the stirrups, Sammie held Susie's hand and talked to her in her beautifully calming, Southern drawl. I placed the speculum in Susie's vagina to see where the cervix sat. There it was, the source of the rotten flesh smell and some of Susie's bleeding: a dark-brown, rough-edged growth in such stark contrast to the smooth, pink, healthy tissue surrounding it. Sammie and I made eye contact. With a subtle nod, I confirmed the diagnosis we'd both been expecting. I quickly obtained biopsies and applied silver nitrate to stop the bleeding from the missing tissue.

After removing the speculum, I conducted a bimanual examination on Susie's pelvic structures, as well as the bones lining her pelvis. Using two fingers, I felt a hard, irregular mass occupying the upper region of Susie's vagina. Placing one hand on her abdomen, I could feel the mass extending to the bones bordering the pelvis on the right side. I knew her tumor had likely spread beyond her cervix and her vagina. It had also cut off the lymph channels draining liquid out of the leg, which explained the swelling. As I finished the exam, Sammie fixed Susie with her warm gaze and told her how happy we were that she had come to see us that day.

The Deadliness of Delaying Care

I left the room as Susie dressed and took a few moments to close my eyes and breathe deeply to compose what I would say. Frankly, I needed to collect my thoughts by clearing the smell from my nostrils and the image of that irregular, oozing, dark mass. I returned to the room. "Susie, I did find a growth at the top of your vagina," I told her. "We won't know for sure until the biopsies return, but I'm worried it may be cancer, and that it may have spread outside your cervix." I stopped. I tried to allow my words to sink in. We sat together in silence. She started to weep. I passed her tissues and reached out to grab her hand. She would not remember most of what I was saying, but I hoped she'd remember my touch.

"Susie, there is treatment for this." Again, I paused, waiting for her to wipe her tears and return my gaze. "I have some excellent partners who specialize in caring for women who have cancer of the cervix. We will get you help." I was thinking that her treatment would mean chemotherapy and radiation, and that because the cancer had spread outside her cervix, her chances for a cure were lower, but still reasonable. When I share such a frightening diagnosis, patients usually ask for information or help, but some can't speak at all because I have confirmed their worst fear, the fear of facing what their instincts already know. This fear can keep people out of doctors' offices altogether. Now that Susie had come to see me, I wanted to do everything I could to keep her coming back and get the treatment that could save her life.

After getting Susie's contact information, I walked her to the waiting area. "I will call you tomorrow to see how you are doing or if you have more questions," I told her. "You do not have to go through this alone."

It was now 1:15 p.m., and afternoon clinic was starting. I slumped onto a stool in a quiet room for a few minutes. I'd encountered something heartbreaking, but sacred. I'd entered a space with Susie where time stopped and everything that came before fell away. I felt complicit, somehow, in Susie's suffering. By uttering the word *cancer*, I'd rewarded a patient for finally seeking care by confirming her worst fear. Tears ran down my cheeks, thinking about Susie, how much her life had changed in the last hour. Did she hear any of the hope I tried to offer?

When she came to the clinic that morning, Susie had reached a crisis point in her health. As I confirmed her fear that "something was really wrong," I, too, echoed those words to myself. *Yes, something is really wrong.* Another patient had received a devastating, possibly terminal diagnosis for a disease I knew to be preventable.

The fact that science had recently deemed her disease preventable offered few reassurances for Susie. She came to a clinic in a country with sophisticated health care systems and resources, and she still ended up with advanced cervical cancer.

No Country Is Immune to the Ravages of Cervical Cancer

Susie's story starts to unpack the uncomfortable truth. Even in the United States, where we can offer vaccines that prevent cervical cancer and tests that can screen and treat for the first possible signs, women face obstacles to lifesaving care. They suffer far more than they should. It's not enough to offer tests, treatments, or vaccines if we are also not addressing the accessibility, financial, and emotional issues that prevent women from using them. In other words, cervical cancer is only as preventable as a country's willingness to provide prevention services *and* to ensure persons with cervixes avail themselves of them. Without the conscientious efforts of caring, committed individuals, health care systems, governments, and global alliances – particularly in the wealthiest nations – the science of prevention simply isn't enough to stop women from dying.

To prevent cervical cancer, we must understand not only how to prevent it, but also *what gets in the way* of preventing it. Part One of this book addresses the scope of this cancer and its economic and social costs. Part Two examines the science of cervical cancer – what causes it, how to prevent it, how to treat it once it occurs, and how being infected with human immunodeficiency virus (HIV) affects cervical cancer's behavior. Part Three delves into the crucial question: What are the social, economic, political, and cultural issues that continue to make this cancer so difficult to stop? Finally, Part Four introduces those devoted to solving the problem of cervical cancer, and how their efforts can inspire us to work alongside them. As it will soon become clear, truly making cervical cancer preventable requires a herculean effort. To meet this goal – that no person with a cervix suffers again from cervical cancer – all of us will need to play a part.

Cervical cancer, of course, is not about numbers or obstacles; it is about people. As such, I have made a point of weaving in the stories of women affected by cervical cancer. Their stories show, in a way that facts and figures can't, just how difficult a journey with cervical cancer can be.

Although I refer to these stories as "women's stories," the term "women" in reference to cervical cancer can be misleading. Cervical cancer happens to persons with cervixes, some of whom may not identify as women. While I often refer to cervical cancer as a "woman's disease" – partly for ease of understanding – it's critical to recognize all genders born with female reproductive organs. Trans men or those born "female" who identify as gay, queer, or nonbinary can be doubly disadvantaged when it comes to seeking cancer care, since they are more likely to face discrimination in any medical environment. They are understandably less likely to pursue a procedure as intimate or uncomfortable as cervical cancer screening. I will talk more about the challenges these individuals face. But for the purposes of this book, the term "women" stands for the cervical cancer prevention needs of all persons with cervixes. I hope readers will offer me grace as I try to navigate an issue that I care about very deeply.

In looking at medical approaches to cervical cancer and global disease spread, I have separated the world into two income-level categories. The World Bank divides countries' gross national incomes into four groups. For the purposes of this book, I have lumped together the top two groups, deeming "higher-income" what the World Bank calls "upper-middle- and high-income" countries and "lower-income" for the "lower-middle- and low-income" countries (Figure 1.1). I've created these two designations partly for ease of argument, but also to show the contrasting abilities for governments to fund health care and delivery systems for their citizens, which includes services for preventing and treating cervical cancer.

No Matter a Country's Wealth – Inequity Is Everywhere

In lower-income countries, the cost of comprehensive cervical cancer prevention and treatment services poses a significant problem; health care budgets in lower-income countries can be less than $100 USD per person per year.[1] With so little to spend on citizens' health, governments must make cervical cancer a priority and direct sufficient resources toward it. These efforts can be stymied not only by financial barriers but also by cultural and social barriers to prevention.

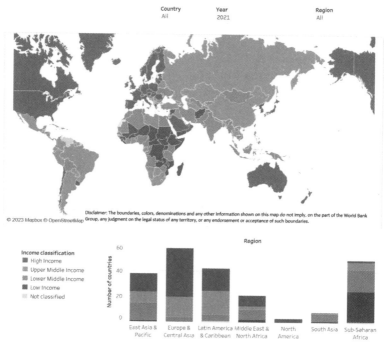

Figure 1.1 World Bank classifications of income levels by country
Source: "The World by Income and Region." The World Bank, accessed Jan 29, 2023. https://datatopics.worldbank.org/world-development-indicators /the-world-by-income-and-region.html

Marginalized communities in higher-income countries face many of the same challenges as lower-income countries, even while wealthy countries spend much more on health care. Underneath the sight line in higher-income countries are women whose poverty level creates a different health care reality – one that is not reflected by the country's World Bank higher-income-level designation. Because society doesn't deem women with low incomes a priority, they suffer from a lack of ready access to the services many of their fellow citizens take for granted. In addition to struggling with personal finances, marginalized women can face – or may solely face – barriers that include stigma, lack of awareness, or specific religious or cultural taboos. While women in lower-income countries typic-ally face far more significant barriers, women in higher-income countries can be affected in a similar way, discouraging them from seeking preventative health care: a "wealthy country problem" that runs counter to many people's expectations.

Despite scarcely resourced countries assuming the burden of disease, these "pockets of inequity" in the developed world explain why this book divides its attention between cancer prevention obstacles in lower-income and higher-income countries. It's astonishing to see such discrepancies in medical care within the same country, and even within smaller geographic regions. Shockingly, U.S. women's diminished access to cervical cancer prevention services can parallel women's experience in parts of Africa: the inability to travel the distance needed to a clinic, the costs that keep care out of reach, or a striking lack of treatment or follow-up care providers, the latter of which causes women with vastly different income levels to compete for the same prevention resources. These are the kinds of factors that make a preventable disease so deadly. Existing social structures suggest a cancer can only be made preventable for those lucky enough to live in the right place and with the money to pay for preventative care.

Because cervical cancer is a global problem, this book features research on cervical cancer prevention across a variety of countries, just as it includes women with access to a diverse range of resources. The book examines obstacles to cervical cancer elimination across diverse geographic locations – countries found in all four hemispheres, some of them densely populated or, conversely, with more sheep than people. I've looked at various economic settings, from countries offering the highest level of medical care to those with scant clinics or hospitals. Of course, I'm most familiar with the U.S. health system where I've based my medical practice. Because the United States offers its citizens a unique, mixed model of private- and public-funded health care, I've compared it with how well women are served in other higher-income countries relying on a publicly funded system, such as the United Kingdom, Canada, and Australia. And while publicly funded health care appears to offer a reliable supply of cervical cancer prevention services, women isolated by geography, finances, or social status aren't necessarily able to take advantage of them.

For women like Susie and Maria, to whom I could offer few words of hope, I hope for this: that by exploring and acknowledging the underlying issues allowing for the continued spread of cervical cancer in both lower- and higher-income countries, we might find a way to erase a disease that continues to rage across the globe; in our failure to help these two women, that we can and will spare others a similar fate.

2 THE VISION

The year was 2003. I was sitting in a University of Washington auditorium packed with 250 people for the announcement of a medical breakthrough. The meeting was partly routine: one of a series of weekly medical educational lectures called "Grand Rounds." Since the 1880s, when the first Grand Rounds were held at the Johns Hopkins University School of Medicine, Grand Rounds has been a much-anticipated event for faculty, residents, and medical students in the United States interested in the latest medical knowledge and scientific innovations. I was keen to hear about progress made in the field of "women's medicine."

At the time, I was a mid-level School of Medicine faculty member, an associate professor in my eleventh year in Obstetrics and Gynecology at the University of Washington. I knew the announcement would be thrilling, with global implications. What I didn't know was that this piece of medical news would ignite a fire inside me – changing my career trajectory – compelling me to align with the fight against cervical cancer worldwide.

The Brash Promise of a Lifesaving Vaccine

I leaned forward in my chair to hear University of Washington epidemiology faculty member Dr. Laura Koutsky, who was well known in the world of human papillomavirus (HPV) research, announce the findings of her four-years-long clinical study. On either side of me was an equally rapt crowd, ranging from third-year medical students to PhD candidates to senior medical professors, diverse in age and experience. From the look of concentration on every face, I could see that we shared a unity of purpose, a laser-like focus on Dr. Koutsky. What she described sounded like a miracle: a new vaccine designed to clear the virus responsible for causing cervical cancer, preventing the deaths of hundreds of thousands of women across the world.

The first clinical trials on this vaccine had just been published in the esteemed *New England Journal of Medicine* – and the results were stunning![1] Between 1998 and 2002, a placebo-controlled vaccine trial conducted in the United States had tested a new HPV-16 vaccine in women aged sixteen to twenty-three. The trial found that the HPV vaccine prevented 100 percent of cancer-causing HPV-16 infections in all women who got the active vaccine. In other words, none – *absolutely zero* – of the nearly 2,400 girls vaccinated went on to develop the persistent HPV-16 infection associated with pre-cancer of the cervix. In marked contrast, 41 of those girls who received the placebo vaccine became infected with HPV-16 (Box 2.1).

I was astounded. The vaccine appeared to virtually eliminate the key virus causing the vast proportion of cervical cancer. The results demonstrated resounding success. As a practitioner who'd spent more than fifteen years screening and treating

---

Box 2.1

You might be wondering why one of the most dangerous types of HPV infections is called "HPV-16." There are actually more than a hundred types of HPV. But only about twelve of them can cause the changes in cervical cells that lead to pre-cancer. These twelve types of HPV are called "oncogenic HPV" or "high-risk HPV" types. Among the oncogenic HPV types, HPV-16 causes the most cervical cancer worldwide, accounting for 50 percent of cases.

women for cervical cancer, I found the implications of a vaccine eradicating this process from the outset to be staggering. While the vaccine was not yet available for broad clinical use, I turned to a few of my colleagues to share my excitement. From the wide eyes and open mouths I saw around me, it was clear we sensed a far brighter landscape ahead in the fight against cervical cancer.

I felt the astonishment settle in: Could the relentless loss of women to cervical cancer be slowed? Perhaps, even stopped?

As part of my work in clinics throughout the United States, my colleagues and I diagnosed new cervical cancer cases several times a year, many of them quite advanced for patients who had received minimal screening. With every diagnosis, I felt the deep grief and internal dissonance of walking with another human's suffering that could easily have been averted. I watched women lose parts of their bodies – sometimes wielding the scalpel myself – and lose not just physical wholeness, but sexual function, bodily functions, self-esteem, hope. I'd seen women's lives stolen from them, their families, their communities.

Dr. Koutsky's astonishing announcement that day morphed into a personal vow for change. As a physician, I was learning about a medical discovery that could potentially save hundreds of thousands of other women's lives across the globe. As a human, I celebrated the chance to see an end to a huge source of human suffering.

I knew I could do more than just imagine this wonderful opportunity. As a doctor, I couldn't wait to be a part of efforts to bring this vaccine to as many young women as possible.

Bracing Myself for a Different Outcome

When I look back on that important day, in some ways, it seems my initial amazement allowed me to be caught up in a bit of a fairy tale. It would be nice to end the story there, to say, "We all lived happily ever after, HPV-infection-free, due to this amazing vaccine." But, of course, the story of cervical cancer has yet to offer the happy ending many of us in the medical community envisioned.

It's now been two decades since that groundbreaking, Grand Rounds announcement, and while the HPV vaccine has gone on to save women's lives, it has failed to garner anywhere near the interest or uptake I'd anticipated. What's more, many lower-income countries, along with marginalized populations within higher-income countries, still struggle to gain access to or convince women to take advantage of cervical cancer screening – the long-standing alternative to vaccination. In the absence of widespread use of cervical cancer prevention measures, the fairy tale has become more of a horror film: not only have recent medical advances failed to halt cervical cancer, but the number of women suffering from cervical cancer is actually increasing.

How could this be?

The numbers don't lie. In 2008, the International Agency for Research on Cancer, a branch of the World Health Organization, reported 530,000 cases of cervical cancer, with nearly 275,000 women dying of the disease. In 2020, the cases of cervical cancer went up to more than 600,000, with more than 340,000 deaths. The organization predicts that in the absence of significant intervention, by 2030, nearly 700,000 women will be diagnosed with cervical cancer and 400,000 of them will die, with analogous increases expected in future. These predictions stand in stark contrast to the euphoria I felt listening to Dr. Koutsky's announcement.

But the escalating rate of cervical cancer cases doesn't provide the whole picture. The ability of the disease to spread so markedly among have-not communities – women in the world's lower-income countries dying in shockingly vast numbers – makes this cancer much harder to stop. Ninety percent of the women who died of cervical cancer in 2020 lived in lower-income countries,[2] largely because these countries lacked the means – and, some would say, the global political clout – to put this preventable medical issue at the top of their health agendas. They're unlikely to do so now without the courageous support of their wealthier counterparts. Cervical cancer has become a disease marked by global inequality.

But what comes as a further shock is the discovery of pockets or regions of higher-income countries with the same cervical cancer rates as some lower-income countries. Many of my patients at Harborview in Seattle, one of the wealthiest cities in the United States, come to us because we offer a relatively rare service: care for women who are, for many reasons, without health insurance. I see patients whose care has been intermittent or radically delayed, their prognoses far worse than other residents with access to world-class health care and the insurance to pay for it. I find it immensely tragic that these terrible inequities stand in the way of preventing cervical cancer in my own relatively privileged country – that even in the United States, cervical cancer remains a disease of inequity.

My fantastical vision of a cervical-cancer-free world has yet to be realized. I've watched economic and political villains threaten and destroy hope; I've watched social and cultural dragons – including underlying beliefs about women's value to society as a whole – torch possibility. I have spent too many years trying to reconcile what should have happened with what is happening. A woman dies of cervical cancer every two minutes, and with that number of deaths growing, I've finally decided to say, "Enough." Enough to reconciling myself to these worldwide realities. Enough suffering. Enough death. I want to move forward, to take down the barriers that prevent the end of a preventable cancer, and to share these findings with people willing to listen, people like you who have picked up this book: Do you share my vision?

I still believe that together we can rewrite the ending to this story gone wrong. That we can collectively offer a conclusion much closer to the one I so naively envisioned sitting in that Grand Rounds auditorium more than twenty years ago.

3 MUST WE ASK WHAT A WOMAN IS WORTH?

On August 24, 2019, on an achingly clear, summer Saturday in Savannah, Georgia, Teolita died of cervical cancer with her mother, Nina, by her side. She was just thirty-eight years old. College-educated, energetic, and caring, a talented writer and ambassador for Cervivor – the high-profile support and advocacy group for cervical cancer sufferers and survivors – Teolita expected to be one of those survivors.* She had been Nina's only child, her mother's world.

I talked with Nina more than a year later from my Seattle office on a gray Monday afternoon in November, the clouds outside my office window heavy and low to the ground. The wintry weather mirrored my emotions as I spoke with Nina over Zoom. Here was a mother who had lost her only daughter to cervical cancer. And here was I, a stranger, asking Nina to relive her daughter's four years of suffering and her own devastating loss. As a mother of adult children, I also felt like an intruder, knowing that in probing Nina about her daughter's encounter with cervical cancer, I would be treading into tender territory.

"We got the news that she had cancer on the day of my mother's birthday," Nina told me. "Teolita adored her grandmother. She did not like one bit having to share the joyous occasion of her grandmother's birthday with this terrible news."

---

* Started by a fellow survivor, Cervivor is a 6,000+ member cervical cancer juggernaut, providing support, education, and advocacy for a global community. Cervivor often uses the color or word teal in their information (e.g., "Teal Tuesday") because cervical cancer is associated with the color teal, and symbolized by teal-colored ribbons (similar to breast cancer being associated with pink). "Color of Cancer Ribbons and Meanings," 2022, accessed March 19, 2023, www.cancerprotalk.com/color-of-cancer-ribbons-and-meanings /#:~:text=Some%20cancer%20ribbons%20are%20multiple%20colors.%20With%2013% 2C000,the%20importance%20of%20early%20detection%20and%20HPV%20prevention

Although Nina's daughter hadn't been experiencing pain, for months, she'd had abnormal bleeding between periods, prompting her to go to the hospital emergency room six months earlier. "They did an ultrasound and told her that she probably had an infection around her [fallopian] tubes and they gave her some antibiotics." But Teolita's bleeding continued, and when a second emergency room visit resulted in the same response, Teolita asked to see a gynecologist.

And that is how Teolita came to have her first Pap smear at thirty-four, a fact Nina deeply regrets. "I think Teolita just did not know she should get Pap smears, and I did not teach her as well as I could have."

My heart broke as I heard Nina's burden – blaming herself for failing to teach her daughter about cervical cancer screening. The truth is that many women don't know the purpose of Pap tests, and many more don't understand their own cervical cancer risks (Box 3.1). As with so many things related to women's bodies and their care, the Pap and other screening tests require tremendously clear, careful, and persistent public communication.

Box 3.1

A Pap smear, Pap, or smear test – "Pap" being short for test developers Dr. George "Papanicolaou" and his wife, Mary (who was his laboratory technician) – is used to detect cervical pre-cancer or cancer. Pap tests take place during a pelvic exam. With the help of a speculum, which holds the sides of the vagina open for visualizing the cervix, a medical provider swabs the cervix using a long, Q-tips cotton swab to gather a broad sample of cervical cells. Trained professionals then evaluate these cervical cells for abnormalities, such as pre-cancer or cancer. If pre-cancer is found, the intention is to treat it as soon as possible. This is what makes Pap smear screening – involving both the testing and, if necessary, the follow-up treatment – a means of preventing cervical cancer. More information about Pap testing and screening for cervical cancer is discussed in Chapter 5.

And information-sharing doesn't pay for the test or make it easily available in everyone's neighborhood. Teolita certainly wasn't the first woman I knew to take her initial screening test well past the recommended age.

A Gynecology Visit Reveals a Dire Prognosis

Teolita's Pap smear revealed abnormalities and she was sent for a colposcopy, a pelvic examination allowing a provider to look for abnormal cells, and if found, to do a biopsy. Teolita asked Nina to join her for the procedure. "Of course I was happy to," Nina said. As Teolita's mother spoke about this day, she looked away from her computer screen, seeming to stare at a distant object. Her facial muscles stiffened, as though gathering strength. "I will never forget the day of the colposcopy," she said in a low, quiet tone. Nina learned from a gynecologist that Teolita had advanced cervical cancer, a diagnosis soon confirmed by a radiation oncologist, who added that Teolita would likely only live another nine to eighteen months.

As Nina spoke, I was momentarily jolted. Imagine what it would be like to bring your child for one simple procedure and hear a terminal prognosis – imagine that. I imagined what this news might be like for me to receive as a mother – learning that I might have only a year or so to spend with one of my precious sons, that I might outlive my own child. In fact, one of my sons had barely survived a car crash a few years before, and my body immediately reverted to the pulsing anguish and choking fear I felt when I first heard the news of his car wreck. It wasn't hard to imagine Nina's pain.

"We did not like that news much," Nina said wryly, and she grew animated as she continued. "We came up with a treatment plan for strong chemotherapy and radiation." After twenty-five radiation and chemotherapy treatments, Teolita enjoyed a brief remission and Nina and her daughter felt hope for her recovery. Teolita had moved to Georgia to be closer to her mother, studying marketing at Savannah State University and working full-time. Despite her cancer diagnosis, Teolita did finish her degree.

"She was so proud of that," her mom told me with a wistful expression.

But her daughter's losses were mounting. "Before her diagnosis, Teolita's life was full of friends and joy – she loved to laugh – and she always had a great deal of energy," Nina recalled. "Initially, her close friends stood by her. But one by one, her friends seemed to move on as she went into treatment." And those who stayed didn't seem to understand what Teolita was going through. "Teolita would go to class and do her job, and people kept telling her, 'You look too good for someone with cancer,' and Teolita used to reply, 'How am I supposed to look?'"

"Teolita would go to class and do her job, and people kept telling her, 'You look too good for someone with cancer,' and Teolita used to reply, 'How am I supposed to look?'"

As I listened to Nina recount her daughter's months of agonizing treatment, it reminded me that during the very time patients most need support, friends may not always be up to the task. Loneliness becomes just another burden for cancer survivors and their caretakers – which was certainly the case for Nina and Teolita. The stigma of cervical cancer – and others' fear of death – represent further cruel features of this disease.

When Teolita discovered Cervivor, however, she became a Cervivor ambassador and made a steady group of new friends. "She found new energy and purpose," Nina recalled. "She wanted to tell everyone to pay attention to their health – and to get screened for cervical cancer." Because Teolita had never had a Pap smear, "her purpose going forward was to make sure to tell as many people as she could."

Determined to make the most of her time, Teolita hosted luncheons, and even a parade, to raise money for and awareness about cervical cancer. She began writing a book about the relationship of human papillomavirus (HPV) to cervical cancer and managed to complete the book's introduction and first chapter before she became too sick to continue. Despite her cancer recurrence and spread, and even throughout her chemotherapy trials, "Teolita tried to keep going, to be strong, to stay hopeful."

As Teolita's condition worsened, Nina became her full-time caregiver. "I just wanted Teolita to feel loved and cared for and to make sure she knew we were going to get through this together," Nina said. "But I did not have any idea she was going to leave me." Eventually, Teolita's doctor told her nothing else could be done. "But he promised her he would not let her be in pain." Nina shut her eyes for a moment. "And she wasn't – Teolita wasn't in any pain. She died in the hospital, in her sleep. I was there at her side."

Since Teolita's passing, Nina has taken on her daughter's mantle as a cervical cancer ambassador. In January 2020, the first cervical cancer awareness month after Teolita died, Nina hosted another fundraising and awareness luncheon. "It was a great success, and we had a lot of fun doing it together," Nina said. "Teolita would have loved it." Nina grew quiet. "But that friend of Teolita's who hosted the luncheon with me, well, she passed away from cervical cancer just two months later, in March of 2020. In fact, of the three who were so close as friends, two have passed now."

"In fact, of the three who were so close as friends, two have passed now."

Nina hopes to finish the book Teolita started and also plans to write a children's book featuring Teolita as the main character. "I just want to honor her and carry on her legacy," Nina said. She sighed. "I never expected to lose her."

Of course – what mother would?

One Heartbreaking Loss Too Many

As I mulled over my conversation with Nina, I grew angry over the abrupt and unjust end to Teolita's life. Not only did Nina lose her daughter, but all of us lost a young woman filled with vibrancy and hope. We lost the contributions Teolita was making, and her contributions yet to come (Figure 3.1).

In fact, we continue to lose the contributions and futures of young women like Teolita. Every year, we lose nearly 4,500 women in the United States and more than 340,000 around the world to cervical cancer. And the brutal truth is that we could prevent nearly every single one of those deaths right now. We have the testing and the treatment. We have a vaccine, a vaccine against cancer!

But tests and treatments cost money. Vaccines cost money. The painstaking public health communication required to overcome reluctance and fear and stigma costs money. As I try to grapple with this reality, I can't help but ask myself the same question every time I deliver a diagnosis to a young woman like Teolita, every time I sit with a mother like Nina and try to explain what likely caused it, every time I hear about another woman dying of a preventable cancer: *What is a woman worth?*

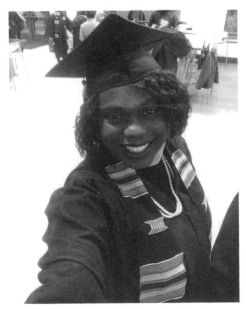

Figure 3.1 Teolita, here overjoyed during graduation from Savannah State University

This is more than just a theoretical question. I really want someone to tell me: What, after all, is a woman truly worth?

In the wake of so many deaths, I want someone to add up all the facts for me and show me how Teolita's life could possibly be deemed not worth saving. I want them to tell me how the lives of more than 340,000 women every year aren't worth saving.

When I ask what women are worth, of course I'm not asking about their intrinsic value, which is easy for us to see in a beloved mother, a precious daughter, a dear friend. As someone who treats cervical cancer, I'm frankly asking a far bigger question of our communities, our systems, our governments, and our global alliances: What is a woman worth to you? What is the price of her life?

This might sound like a crass question. But in the context of preventing death from cervical cancer, it's important to quantify women's worth, because prevention costs money. The price tag associated with vaccines, screening, and early treatment of this disease requires the political will to make cervical cancer resources and infrastructure a health care priority that receives sufficient funding among competing interests. Political will is always entwined with economic demands. A woman's worth tragically hangs somewhere in the balance.

Investing in Women Makes Good Economic Sense

We need only scan the globe to find easy evidence that women are not yet deemed a worthwhile investment. In countries of sub-Saharan Africa, like Niger, or in India or Bangladesh, what does the practice of child marriage – where young girls are married to older men with multiple prior sexual partners – say about a girl's worth? In regions of the United States that require a woman on minimum wage to travel five hours by car to reach a health care provider offering an affordable Pap smear or a sliding-fee colposcopy, what are we saying about how much that woman is worth? Few would deny that preventing the deaths of these women and girls doesn't make emotional sense. But until that sentiment trans-lates into public policy and reliable, affordable health care plans equally accessible to all women, lofty ideas will not save lives.

To Nina, Teolita was "worth everything." To a seven-year-old whose mother dies of cervical cancer, life will never be the same. To a young woman whose cervical cancer robs her and her partner of the ability to have children, what wouldn't they pay to have that back? These losses are devastating, next to impossible to quantify. But they will need to be quantified so that communities, governments, systems, and global partner-ships understand the price being paid every time a woman is diagnosed with or dies of cervical cancer.

And so, I ask the question again: what is a woman worth?

When health economists look at spending money on health care interventions, they measure and compare the "worth" of these interventions in terms of their cost and return on invest-ment. The World Health Organization's health economy team has calculated that for lower-income countries, accounting for 90 percent of cervical cancer cases, every dollar invested in cervical cancer screening through 2050 will return an estimated $3.20 USD to that country's economy.[1] And these calculations are only based on women's increasing participation in the workforce over the next thirty years. They don't account for the countless hours of unpaid labor critical to families, commu-nities, and economies: household management, childcare, care of the elderly, and numerous volunteer commitments. When these unpaid contributions of women's labor are factored into the calculation of "worth," a total of $26 USD is returned to a country. In other words, every dollar spent on prevention promises a return on investment of $26 USD directly back into a community – a prudent investment, to be sure.

In other words, every dollar spent on prevention promises a return on investment of $26 USD directly back into a community – a prudent investment, to be sure.

WHO senior health economist Dr. Raymond Hutubessy, who led the cost–benefit analysis for lower-income countries investing in cervical cancer screening, sees this sort of dollars-and-cents information as a means for governments to make concrete decisions around prevention spending. He believes, as I do, that spending on cervical cancer prevention is a bargain: the economic return on investing in a preventable cancer far outweighs the initial expense. "I was surprised at just how cost-effective cervical cancer prevention is," Dr. Hutubessy told me in 2020, and again in 2022. "Resources are not infinite. But spending money on cervical cancer prevention offers such excellent benefits for a country."

"I was surprised at just how cost-effective cervical cancer prevention is. Resources are not infinite. But spending money on cervical cancer prevention offers such excellent benefits for a country."

This reasoning offers the rationale for continuing to talk about the cost of cervical cancer in dollar amounts: over and above the dismal, incalculable loss of human life – the real costs of screening, testing, treatment, and prevention. Because if we're ever going to eliminate a cancer that needn't exist, we'll have to understand the financial benefits of that effort.

Looking Past the Numbers

In my practice, I care for humans. I treat their bodies, which are part and parcel to their hearts, their minds, their relationships. And I'm a mother, a daughter, and a friend, who loves the women in my life and values them far beyond price. I'm also an avid reader and I know the power of stories. Numbers may be important, but they will never fully convey the suffering of my cervical cancer patients, and price tags will never galvanize us to the fight ahead – the elimination of a cancer worldwide – the way human stories will.

And so, we'll talk about what a woman is worth outside of economies. We would never ask a mother like Nina to give us an actual price tag for her daughter's life, because her value was beyond measure. The "worth" of a daughter to a mother (or a mother to a daughter, a sister to a sister, a spouse to her partner, a friend to a friend) is something we can all feel and connect with. We can put ourselves in Nina's place and readily sympathize with what it might feel like to bury a daughter before she turns forty – the injustice of it, the feeling that "life is not supposed to be this way. I am not supposed to be the one burying my child. My child was supposed to live longer than me." We can imagine the deep ache, as well, of losing a life partner – someone we've chosen to travel through life's adventures and joys and struggles with – to this cruel disease. A partner no longer sitting in her favorite chair at evening's end. We can even imagine – as much as we don't want to – what it might be like for a seven-year-old, or a fifteen-year-old, or a twenty-year-old to lose a mother, the one who advocates for them and believes in them in a way no one else does. That protective Mama-bear, no longer present. And those ripples of loss that extend beyond a woman's immediate or extended family. Those of us who have lost a friend to death of any sort know that these losses are felt for years; that person will hold a place in our hearts for life.

A woman's "worth" doesn't end with family and friends, either. Women are the social glue and fabric of our societies. They are the backbone of most volunteer organizations; they run school parent associations and medical volunteer groups and form the ranks of endless civic, arts, and nonprofit organizations that feed their communities in myriad ways. Women run voting organizations, organize clothing drives, and take food to neighbors in need. In lower-income countries, women are often integral to the informal economies that literally keep families fed; in countries where men are forced to migrate for work, whole villages of women remain behind to carry on every aspect of life: work, farming, education, child-rearing. To measure the worth of women to their communities shouldn't be difficult; it's hard to imagine the world functioning without them.

And yet – these valuable women are dying, by the hundreds of thousands. We can talk about the grief and sadness of losing a woman, and we can create strategies about how to address it, but I also want to look inside – and invite you to do so as well – to ask yourself these questions: *What is a woman really worth to us? And how will we show that? And what will we ask of our communities, our governments, and the world to fight to save them?*

If we're ever going to actually see the elimination of cervical cancer – a cancer that is already preventable – then we're going to have to really dig deep and ask ourselves and others those questions, and when we do, I hope we will all say *Enough! Women are worth everything we can give them.*

Part Two
The Science behind Cervical Cancer

4 THE DANGEROUS CLOUT OF A SEXUALLY TRANSMITTED VIRUS

In 1983, scientists made the brilliant discovery that the human papillomavirus (HPV) was the source of cervical cancer – and through the development of the HPV vaccine gave the world a means to squelch it.[1] Forty years later, surprisingly few members of the general public know how to control HPV, because they don't automatically link it to cervical cancer. As a doctor, I routinely come across patients with little understanding of HPV infections or their deadly significance. Their lack of understanding about HPV concerns me deeply. This sexually transmitted virus poses a significant risk to female reproductive health and global efforts to do away with cervical cancer.

As a gynecologist who routinely screens for cervical cancer, it's my job to educate patients about HPV and preventing cervical cancer – and I'm eager to share the news. Persons with cervixes who understand HPV become empowered keepers of their reproductive systems, promoting good health and well-being. And, when I share facts around HPV, I lay the groundwork for my patients to embrace cervical cancer prevention through the HPV vaccine and screening the cervix for cancer.

What's more, promoting a thorough understanding of HPV and cervical cancer prevention chips away at the stigma of acquiring this virus. Because HPV is sexually transmitted – and most cultures carry powerful moral judgments about sexually transmitted infection – the "HPV-positive" label can confer a heavy emotional burden. It essentially implies someone has been "caught" having sex, whether frequently or infrequently or even with multiple partners. Patients labeled "HPV-positive" feel embarrassed, ashamed, and even afraid before they begin thinking about the steps to preventing cervical cancer. My conversations with these patients need to consider their sensitivities. This is possibly my one-and-only chance to address their worries while furthering their understanding about this stealth virus – one vulnerable person with a cervix at a time.

Jennifer, a twenty-six-year-old and one of my HPV-positive patients with a limited understanding of the virus and cervical cancer, expressed terror over her initial HPV-DNA test results. I moved quickly to put her mind at ease. It's been my experience that patients armed with knowledge are in a far better position to prevent cancer than those who are inundated with fear-fueled misunderstanding and misinformation.

HPV Is More Common Than You Think

I was working in my clinic in Seattle one Thursday in May. As I scrolled through messages in my patient care inbox, Jennifer's name popped up right away. She'd sent me three messages. The first one, from early in the day, noted that her Pap smear results had come back atypical. "It also says I have this 'high-risk, HPV-DNA-positive' result," she wrote. "What does that mean?"

Four hours later, Jennifer had sent me another message: "Can I ever get rid of this? Who gave this to me?"

Finally, just a couple of hours after the second message, I saw Jennifer's third message. This one let me know her underlying fear: "Dr. Eckert, am I going to get cancer?"

As I read the escalating tone of these messages, I could tell that Jennifer was only growing more worried as the day wore on. I wish I could say her sense of urgency was unusual, but it's not. Jennifer's concerns were – and are – valid. And they're all too common. Ever since 2003, when our Seattle clinic began using HPV-DNA tests for women who'd received slightly abnormal Pap smear results, I've received many such panicked messages from patients. HPV-DNA tests are highly effective: they rely on objective lab findings rather than the subjective judgment of a pathologist, so they're more medically precise than standard Pap smears. However, while HPV-DNA tests can provide a clearer picture of the likelihood of developing pre-cancer, they also detect the presence of HPV, introducing the added element of stigma.

From a patient's perspective, the combination of "high-risk," "positive," and "abnormal Pap smear" – terms that might show up on a cervical screening report combining HPV-DNA test data with Pap smear results – is a scary triad to read or hear over the phone. I was not surprised to learn Jennifer was worried.

I moved into a private room where I could shut the door, ruminating over how I could dispel Jennifer's panic while urging her to pursue the follow-up testing she needed. I called her back.

"Hi Jennifer, it's Dr. Eckert. Is this a good time for you?" She asked me to wait while she found a private room for chatting. I heard the patter of her footsteps, and then the shutting of a door.

"Okay, I'm ready now," she said.

Trying to convey warmth, I told Jennifer I wanted her to have all the facts so she could interpret her results. "I want to allay your greatest concern first. Human papillomavirus, or HPV, is incredibly common. But having HPV does not mean that you have cancer."

"Human papillomavirus, or HPV, is incredibly common. But having HPV does not mean that you have cancer."

I heard a pause, so I continued. "To give you an idea of how common HPV is – by the time a woman has had three sexual partners, more than fifty percent of the time, she'll have an HPV infection.[2] Also, eighty percent of adults will have HPV in their lifetimes."[3]

"Really? HPV is that common?" Jennifer said.

"Yes, absolutely. And, there are actually more than a hundred types of HPV. But only about twelve of them can cause changes in the cells covering the cervix that might lead to pre-cancer, and then, possibly, cancer," I told her. These twelve types of HPV are called 'oncogenic' or 'high-risk HPV' types."[*]

"But doesn't 'oncogenic' mean cancer?'" Jennifer said, her voice rising. "I thought you said I didn't have cancer?"

"No, Jennifer – you do not have cancer. When a report says 'high-risk HPV-DNA-positive' with atypical cells, this means you have an infection with one of the twelve high-risk types of HPV. It means we want to follow your results more carefully. It does not mean that you're necessarily going to get cervical cancer."

"Okay. That's good. But how can I get rid of HPV?" These were the words I was hoping to hear, since explaining how to manage HPV would give me a chance to settle Jennifer's fears while steering her toward preventing cervical cancer.

HPV Doesn't Always Equal Cancer

"Well, the good news is that our body usually gets rid of the HPV infection by itself," I told her. "The virus slips in under the layers of the cervical lining, and it can stay there, unnoticed, because it doesn't cause any symptoms. Our immune systems can fight off the infection caused by the virus, and the HPV will stop replicating. If the virus is not replicating, it doesn't cause any harm. Over ninety percent of HPV infections will resolve within two years – often sooner."[3]

"In your case, Jennifer, we'll want to give your body time to get rid of the virus before your next test. So, we wait one year. Then we'll do another HPV-DNA test and another Pap smear to see if the HPV-DNA is still present."

"How do I know who gave this to me?" she asked. I hear this question a lot, but it can be hard to answer. Because HPV is so

---

[*] Currently, twelve HPV types are defined as high-risk (oncogenic) and cause cancer in humans (types 16, 18, 31, 33, 35, 39, 45, 51, 52, 56, 58, 59); type 68 is classified as probably causing cancer. Type HPV-16 is the most oncogenic. IARC Working Group on the Evaluation of Carcinogenic Risks to Humans, "Biological Agents," *IARC Monogr Eval Carcinog Risks Hum* **100**, no. Pt B (2012): 1–441. www.ncbi.nlm.nih.gov/pubmed/23189750

common and doesn't cause symptoms, it was hard to tell who might have exposed Jennifer to HPV.

"While the virus could have come from your most recent partner," I told her, "it could also have come from a previous partner."

"Should my partner get tested? Should I use a condom now?" she asked, both questions I would go on to hear almost every time I told a woman she had HPV. Jennifer happened to have a male partner, so I told her we didn't have an HPV test to offer men. "We do not have an HPV screening test widely used for men. Relative to HPV's impact on the cervix, pre-cancer or cancer of the penis from HPV is much more rare. Additionally, exactly how to screen men for HPV, and what to do with the results, is not clear." If my patient had a female partner, I would simply have told her that her partner should protect herself by seeking regular cervical cancer screening. Regarding condoms, I told Jennifer that any skin-to-skin genital contact can transfer HPV, including skin not covered by a condom. Condoms do decrease HPV transmission by about 60 percent,[4] but even with using condoms all of the time, HPV can be shared between partners. So, while my patients like Jennifer may feel stigmatized by having HPV, I hope to offer some reassurance by conveying just how common this virus is, and that even 100 percent condom use does not prevent catching it from a partner.

As I reminded Jennifer of the importance of a repeat HPV-DNA test and Pap smear in one year's time – key steps in preventing cervical cancer – I asked her one final question. "By the way, are you a smoker?"

"No, I'm not," she said. "Why do you ask?"

"Smoking tobacco makes it harder for your body to get rid of the HPV infection," I told her. "I would say 'quit smoking' if you're a smoker."

After checking with Jennifer to make sure I'd answered all of her questions, I hung up and took advantage of a rare private moment to think about our conversation. It occurred to me just how much more information I had to offer about HPV than I'd had in 1991, when I'd first started practicing as an obstetrician and gynecologist.

In 1992, University of Washington faculty member Dr. Laura Koutsky would lead a landmark study[5] showing that 28 percent of women with a new, high-risk HPV infection developed pre-cancer within two years, half of which came from a particular type of HPV: HPV-16. This study was one of the first to follow women over time and demonstrate the direct link between high-risk HPV infections and pre-cancer.

But as I now tell my patients like Jennifer, this doesn't mean that persons with cervixes who acquire HPV-16 or other high-risk HPV types will get pre-cancer, because 85 to 90 percent of the time, the body clears the HPV infection. Even when HPV causes pre-cancer, the body can still get rid of it before it becomes cancer. Given the frequency of HPV infections, the body's ability to clear a dangerous virus is terrific news.

However, the presence of high-risk HPV is still worrisome. When a patient's screening tests detect HPV-DNA, follow-up testing is critical.

So, when does HPV-DNA in the cervix pose the greatest risk? Studies have associated "persistent HPV infections" – infections of the same HPV type for at least twelve months – with surface changes on the cervix leading to cancer. That's why I urge patients such as Jennifer to repeat their HPV-DNA tests a year later to ensure their HPV infections haven't persisted. Since persistent HPV infections with high-risk HPV types are so much more worrisome, it's important to understand what factors contribute to persistent HPV. As I discussed with Jennifer, smoking is one of those factors. But perhaps the most noteworthy factor in HPV persistence is an altered immune system, especially for patients with human immunodeficiency virus (HIV).

Persons with cervixes diagnosed with HIV have a significantly harder time clearing HPV infections, making them six times more likely to contract cervical cancer than those without HIV.[6] But patients who take immune-system-suppressing medications (immunosuppressants), such as medications required after organ transplants to prevent organ rejection, also have altered immune systems, which make them more vulnerable to HPV infections. Women who require immunosuppressants for autoimmune health conditions, such as severe arthritis, lupus, or inflammatory bowel disease, are at higher risk of developing cervical cancer if they contract a high-risk HPV infection and are at increased risk of other HPV-related consequences, such as genital warts.

Stigma Gets in the Way of Prevention

Just as women living with HIV face terrible stigma, which can interfere with their ability to access timely or suitable care, the stigma associated with an HPV infection can discourage women from talking about it with their doctors or others. Jennifer expressed such concerns when she asked me how to tell her partner she had HPV.

Women who develop pre-cancer or cancer from an HPV infection often feel shameful and blame themselves for their disease. These feelings present another barrier to seeking lifesaving follow-up care. Many patients have told me over the years that one of the worst features of contracting HPV is feeling humiliated or judged about getting HPV from having sex or being treated for cervical pre-cancer. Nearly every cervical cancer sufferer I interviewed for this book told me she felt shamed by the stigma of HPV and cervical cancer, despite the fact that most of us will have an HPV infection at some point in our lives. If anything, these women need extra emotional support. It makes little sense to alienate people fighting cancer by judging how and why they might have gotten the disease.

Perhaps one of the cruelest ironies around HPV stigma comes from blaming sexual assault victims for acquiring HPV. Statistics indicate that one in six women will be sexually assaulted. Researchers have yet to study how often HPV is transmitted through sexual assault. However, unlike other sexually transmitted infections, such as gonorrhea or chlamydia, which are prevented by giving antibiotics to sexual assault victims, there is no way to prevent a sexually assaulted woman from being exposed to HPV.

I remember speaking with one patient after she'd received test results of an abnormal Pap smear with the presence of high-risk HPV. "Do you think I could have gotten this from when I was sexually assaulted eight months ago?" she asked me. I could offer her no real answer, only words of comfort as I watched her eyes fill with tears. The way she immediately cast her eyes downward bore witness to her pain and shame.

In working with patients who come to our clinic from lower-income countries, I have also watched a woman's inferior social status and marriage at a young age become risk factors for acquiring HPV and subsequent disease. Beena came to see me when she was thirty-four and recently relocating from Gambia. In exchange for three goats, her father had married Beena to one of his friends when she was just fifteen. Her husband was fifty-one. Beena did not want this marriage, and her husband did not treat her well. When he later died of a stroke, Beena was able to leave Gambia with her three children and join her sister, living in Seattle.

Beena was shy, but her warm grin lit up the room. I performed her first-ever Pap smear and pelvic examination. When Beena's Pap smear results indicated cervical pre-cancer, I told her about the role of HPV. She told me that she'd only had one sexual partner in her life, but she knew that her husband had had many partners. As we discussed her need and options for treatment, she said it was good she no longer lived in her village, because any problem with her womb would be "my fault."

Unfortunately, the idea of "fault" in connection to acquiring HPV is not unique to Beena, or to Gambia, as Jennifer and so many of my other patients have expressed to me in my years of practice. Beena's and Jennifer's stories demonstrate just how challenging it can be to negotiate the news of having HPV, and how much fear and stigma can get in the way of seeking the care necessary to prevent cervical cancer.

This is why the simple act of giving my patients information is so empowering – even liberating.

As I help my patients realize just how common an HPV infection is and what an important role it plays in detecting cervical cancer, my patients and I can proactively care for their cervixes. My key message: most HPV infections do clear, but for those that don't, it's vital to get regular and recommended follow-up tests. If HPV persists and becomes pre-cancer, then it can still be treated – the sooner, the better.

My key message: most HPV infections do clear, but for those that don't, it's vital to get regular and recommended follow-up tests. If HPV persists and becomes pre-cancer, then it can still be treated – the sooner, the better.

The good news about HPV is that we know what it is, how to test for it, how to treat it, and how to prevent it from causing cervical cancer. The more we spread the word about just how common HPV is, the more we reduce the power of blame and stigma and relegate them to the dust heap where they belong.

5   THE POWER OF PREVENTION

All women remember their first pelvic examination and Pap test. I definitely remember mine.

I was twenty-one. It was July of 1983, and I was one month away from my first year at medical school. I decided that going for a pelvic exam was the responsible thing to do. I would soon be inundated with course work. It was time to get my first Pap smear out of the way. Nervously, I booked my appointment.

We'd had our family physician for more than a decade. He'd been the one to swab my throat to test for strep, the one who'd treated my childhood ear infections. I felt comfortable with him, but despite that comfort and my general knowledge of medicine, I found my first Pap smear intrusive and unwelcoming.

As I waited for my doctor to come in, I sat on the paper sheet that covered the examination table and crinkled with each movement. The room was cold, more noticeable while I was half-naked, with only a sheet covering my bottom half. When the doctor and nurse entered, they asked me to slide my bare bottom to the edge of the table, lie back, and place my feet in a pair of "stirrups." Stirrups – the round, metal foot holders on rods extending from the exam table – symbolize vulnerability. While a patient's legs are suspended in stirrups, her bare thighs naturally splay open, exposing her genital area for examination. *No wonder they keep those stirrups hidden below the table*, I thought to myself. *Better not to know what you're in for in advance.* As I stared at the long, glaring row of fluorescent ceiling lights, I heard the doctor say, "Just let your knees fall apart." Oh. My. Word.

Forty years later, I can close my eyes and immediately go back to those unpleasant feelings. It was embarrassing to be unclothed in this frog-leg position, my body on display to this man from whom I had asked career advice while thinking about going to med school. I realized he was a professional. But I could not overcome the jarring, cold metal speculum being placed into my vagina. As my doctor gathered a sample for the Pap smear, I cringed at the scratchy, pinching, cotton Q-tip sliding around my cervix in a full circle. I felt invaded and intruded upon.

In talking with other women about Pap tests, I've heard them express similar feelings. I know I'm not alone. Let's be honest: no one *wants* to sign up for cervical cancer screening with a pelvic examination. No one *wants* to lie half-naked on an exam table for a speculum examination. Yet somehow, I followed the message to go get screened anyway.

As someone who grew up in a relatively affluent community in the United States, I'd learned that having cervical cancer screening – essentially, getting a Pap smear – was important for taking care of myself. When I studied medicine, I was grateful for that prompting, and yes, even for my screenings: disagreeable, but invaluable in sparing me a cancer that might otherwise go undetected.*

Screening tests like these have been one of the mainstays to saving lives from cervical cancer since their inception in the 1940s.[1] Pap tests may be uncomfortable, even jarring, but they are highly effective. The Pap smear screening test represents only one way to prevent deaths from cervical cancer. In fact, even though hundreds of thousands of women a year die worldwide from cervical cancer, most of these deaths can be prevented with timely cervical cancer screening. If pre-cancer is detected, ongoing treatment and follow-up can halt the progression to cancer. And, if cancer is found early, treatment can lead to a cure. Add to this the uniquely proficient HPV vaccine for

---

* Some cervical cancer screening sites may allow patients to request a female provider.

preventing cancer, and no women at all need to die of cervical cancer.

It seems bold to declare that the vast majority of cervical cancer deaths are preventable – and yet, it's true. In the medical community, the three key interventions for preventing cervical cancer are called "primary," "secondary," and "tertiary" pillars. In ideal circumstances – typically, in higher-income countries – persons with cervixes have access to each of these three pillars. People living in lower-income countries, however, usually have far fewer medical options available to them, including the three pillars that prevent cervical cancer deaths.

Because HPV is responsible for 99 percent of cervical cancer, early HPV vaccinations are the primary pillar. These vaccinations won't allow the most dangerous types of HPV to infect the cervix. Cervical cancer screening to detect and treat pre-cancer of the cervix before it becomes cancer is the secondary pillar. Screening includes tests for pre-cancer abnormalities, such as Pap smears or HPV-DNA testing, and removal of pre-cancer abnormalities. Early treatment for cervical cancer is the third or tertiary pillar of prevention. Because this cancer is slow growing in most women, if it's found early enough, the right treatment can cure it. At this stage, using early follow-up treatment to save lives makes it a form of prevention.

Timing is everything when it comes to saving lives. Girls as young as nine and up to age fourteen are advised to get the HPV vaccine, and screening and treatment for pre-cancer for women start as early as twenty-one, but usually begin somewhere between twenty-five and thirty (Box 5.1). The World Health Organization has developed guidelines and recommendations regarding the ideal ages and frequency for taking advantage of these three prevention pillars. The WHO rationale for these interventions is based on decades of data showing the typical onset of an HPV infection, cervical pre-cancer, and cervical cancer across all higher- and lower-income countries, as well as lower-income regions within higher-income countries.

While the WHO recommends women in many lower-income countries or regions start screening for cervical cancer at thirty,

---

Box 5.1

The HPV vaccine can be given to those older than fifteen, and some countries have approved offering the vaccine up to age forty-five. However, the HPV vaccine will not cure an existing HPV infection; it will only protect against a new infection. While the vaccine is safe to receive at any age, it offers fewer disease-prevention benefits for those who've already been exposed to high-risk types of HPV. Still, even if one type of HPV is present in the cervix, the vaccine can offer protection from other HPV types that may be introduced through sexual contact with new partners.

Box 5.2

Cervical cancer is almost nonexistent for women younger than twenty-one, and it only rarely occurs for those under twenty-five. Historically, screening recommendations have gradually changed to reflect the typical onset of cervical cancer as well as the body's ability to naturally clear HPV infections – particularly at a young age. These changes also take into account the potential problem of overtreating women for HPV infections that otherwise would have resolved on their own.

---

many higher-income countries typically start screening earlier (Figure 5.1). In the United States, Europe, Canada, and Australia, for example, women get their first screening tests at around twenty-five. Doctors in the United States used to begin screening at eighteen, which then became twenty-one – the age I had my first Pap (Box 5.2). As more sensitive and sophisticated screening tests come available, such as HPV-DNA tests, and HPV vaccination becomes more common, women in affluent

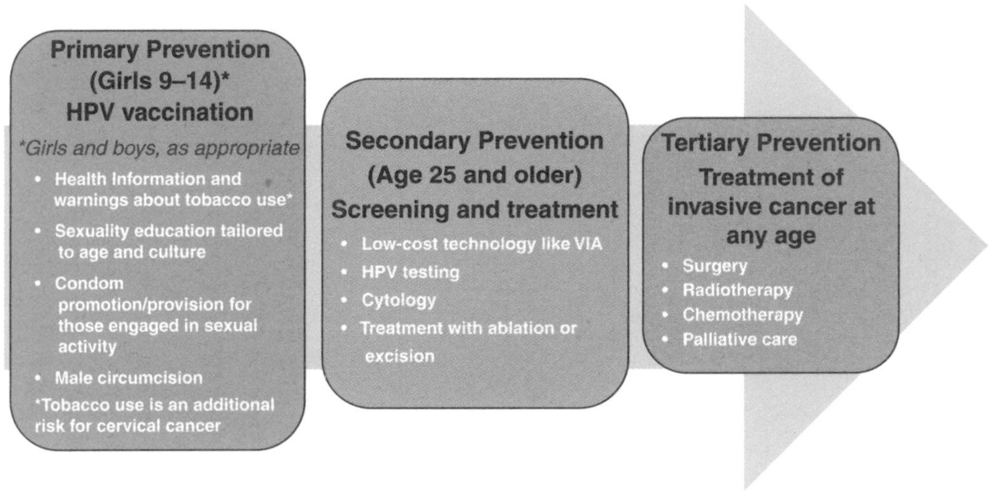

Figure 5.1 Prevention strategies and recommended age interventions against cervical cancer. VIA = Visual Inspection with Acetic Acid

Source: Adapted from *Global Strategy to Accelerate the Elimination of Cervical Cancer as a Public Health Problem*. Geneva: World Health Organization, 2020. https://www.who.int/publications/i/item/9789240014107

countries are being told to get their first screening tests done at a later age.[2]

New technology hasn't changed the importance of treating pre-cancer when it's found. To increase the likelihood of detecting pre-cancer, women need to be screened at recommended intervals up to age sixty-five. Screening requires commitment, but it saves lives. According to a 2018 U.S.-based study conducted over thirty years, an estimated half-million cases of cervical cancer were prevented by women taking part in regularly recommended Pap screening tests.[3]

Treatment – the third pillar of prevention – is in the "prevention" category, because the goal of stopping cervical cancer has now morphed into preventing women from dying of it. Relying on treatment to keep women alive is far more complicated, expensive, and invasive. Ideally, women who receive the first two pillars of vaccination and screening turn only rarely to the third pillar. Of course, regular screening increases the chances of cancer being found early, when treatment has the best chance of succeeding.

Despite the effectiveness of these three pillars, the bitter truth for many persons with cervixes is a profound lack of access to prevention measures. This translates into tragic circumstances: without vaccination or screening, women are left – and only if they're lucky – with the final pillar: treatment of cancer once it's found. But even when treatment is available, cervical cancer is typically found too late to offer a significant chance of survival, because cervical cancer often is without symptoms in its early stages.

In other words, eliminating deaths from cervical cancer is only possible when women have comprehensive and consistent access to all three pillars.

HPV Vaccines Are Fearsome Cancer Killers

In layman's terms, the HPV vaccine is a gold star insurance policy: it offers maximum protection against cervical cancer before exposure to HPV – essentially when persons with cervixes are young or before they've had sex for the first time. The vaccine also creates a stronger immune response in girls under fifteen. Nine to fourteen is considered the ideal age range for receiving the HPV vaccine, because it bolsters younger immune systems before HPV exposure.

In addition to offering spectacular protection against cervical cancer, the HPV vaccine prevents a wide range of other cancers. HPV-16 is responsible for a large proportion of vulvar and vaginal cancers in women and anal and throat cancers in men and women (Figure 5.2). When you consider that HPV causes 35,000 cancers every year in the United States alone, the potency of the HPV vaccine is nothing short of amazing.[*]

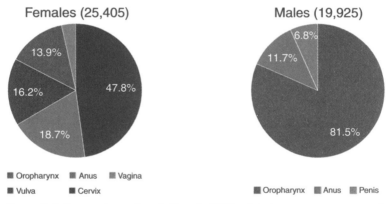

Figure 5.2 Comparison of male/female HPV-related cancers over a year in the United States.
Source: "Cancers Associated with Human Papillomavirus, United States—2013–2017." U.S. Cancer Statistics Data Briefs, Centers for Disease Control and Prevention. Updated September 2020, accessed Jan 29, 2023. https://www.cdc.gov/cancer/uscs/about/data-briefs/no18-hpv-assoc-cancers-UnitedStates-2013-2017.htm.

---

[*] The earliest types of HPV vaccines focused on preventing the two HPV types most commonly associated with cervical cancer: HPV-16 and HPV-18. These two types account for 70 percent of cervical cancer cases. In 2014, the U.S. Food and Drug Administration (FDA) approved another HPV vaccine. This new vaccine, Gardasil 9 (sometimes written HPV9), protects against HPV-16 and HPV-18 and five additional high-risk HPV types (31, 33, 45, 52, and 58), resulting in protection against about 90 percent of cervical cancer. E. Petrosky, J. A. Bocchini, Jr., S. Hariri, *et al.*, "Use of 9-Valent Human Papillomavirus (HPV) Vaccine: Updated HPV Vaccination Recommendations of the Advisory Committee on Immunization Practices," *MMWR Morb Mortal Wkly Rep* **64**, no. 11 (March 27, 2015): 300–4. www.ncbi.nlm.nih.gov/pubmed/25811679

Thanks to the HPV vaccine – and for people and countries that can afford it – we have a nearly unparalleled prevention measure for cervical cancer, along with many other deadly cancers.[4,5] But because so many countries are waiting to get their hands on the vaccine, we've yet to put its miraculous properties to the test. A wide variety of economic, political, and social obstacles still stand in the way of unleashing this cancer-destroying weapon worldwide.

Keep in mind that this astonishing vaccine is a relatively "recent" invention. The HPV vaccine wasn't available in the United States or other higher-income countries until 2006, meaning millions of women born too late to avail themselves of the vaccine got left behind. (U.S. women who turned twenty-seven, for instance, the year the vaccine was approved – and their compatriots born before 1980 – were "too old" to meet the country's targeted nine to twenty-six age range. Millions more didn't make the cut in other higher-income countries, depending on vaccine availability and their designated age ranges.) In lower-income countries, the vaccine was offered to far fewer women – either years after its introduction or not at all.

Considering the number of women left unvaccinated and unprotected, the vaccine alone cannot be deemed a panacea. Disease elimination must rely heavily on screening and follow-up measures. Screening remains a proven and well-known prevention pillar, and in some countries, it's the *only* available pillar.

Screening a Reliable Ally against Cancer

All women need secondary prevention for cervical cancer, even those who have received the HPV vaccine. Today's HPV vaccines protect against 70 to 90 percent – but not 100 percent – of cervical cancer. Women who've been vaccinated must keep going for Pap tests or other similar screening tests, and then seek medical follow-up and treatment for "positive" test results.

In North American and European countries offering widespread Pap smear testing, cervical cancer rates have fallen dramatically. Australia, which offers a publicly funded medical system and vast support for prevention programs, is on track to be first to eliminate cervical cancer by the year 2035. (Yes – you heard that right! Cervical cancer elimination can be done!)

The success of screening and treatment for pre-cancer, or secondary prevention, in the higher-income world contrasts sharply with regions that can't afford or have yet to introduce widely accessible screening and follow-up measures – including a number of countries in Africa, some South American countries, and parts of Southeast Asia. In these countries, cervical cancer rates are increasing. Yet, the benefits of cervical cancer screening are clear: in most cases, regular testing can effectively do away with this disease, even without HPV vaccination.

Secondary prevention works well because cervical pre-cancer and cancer are slow growing. When HPV infects a cervix, HPV takes months to years before possibly turning into pre-cancer, and several years to become cancer. Among regularly screened women, pre-cancer is more likely to be detected and successfully treated during this latency period. Of course, cancer is still a wild card; not all cancer behaves "as it should." Cancer incidence varies widely according to patient age, medical history, and other aggravating factors. The cervical cancer sufferers featured in this book include those who followed screening recommendations and still got cervical cancer. Their experiences remind us that despite this cancer's typical slow growth, it's critical to adhere to a doctor-recommended screening schedule.

What's more, the word *screening* sometimes fails to consider its two distinct steps: testing *and* follow-up. Screening tests alone will not reduce cancer. Should that test reveal abnormalities or pre-cancer, it *must* be followed by early treatment. Indeed, the success of secondary prevention for cervical cancer depends on follow-up care – the extra steps that countries lacking significant reproductive health budgets for women don't automatically provide, steps women might overlook when they haven't received clear and consistent messages about the need for follow-up.

Follow-up treatment typically involves removing pre-cancerous tissue using relatively minor procedures known as "ablation" or "excision."* These procedures are done when the pre-cancer is in its latency period, before it has a chance to turn into cancer. Occasionally, patients with cervical pre-cancer require a "cone biopsy" to remove a large or particularly serious pre-cancerous abnormality. In countries or regions with access to the right equipment and trained providers, these treatments are 90 percent effective in preventing pre-cancer from becoming cancer. Treatment for cervical pre-cancer, whether it's by ablation or excision, is far less arduous than the treatment needed for cancer once it appears. Compared with cancer treatment, treatment for pre-cancer is markedly cheaper, requires much less time off work, and creates less economic hardship. Most importantly, treating cervical pre-cancer can mean avoiding the permanent, life-altering consequences that can accompany cervical cancer treatment (more about this in Chapter 6). So, while treatment with ablation or excision presents challenges, it is worth the effort and money to treat the disease at the pre-cancer stage.

During the two years after treatment for pre-cancer, patients need frequent screening for possible recurrences. This post-treatment vigilance challenges countries already struggling to provide comprehensive care, as well as patients unable to access

---

* Ablation involves freezing pre-cancerous tissue using a "cryotherapy probe," or by using a heat-based technique called "thermocoagulation." Ablation procedures may cause cramping, but are relatively pain free and performed without local anesthesia. Ablations offer an additional advantage to pre-cancer sufferers who lack access to sophisticated medical care in lower-income countries, since these procedures do not require physicians. They can instead be performed by well-trained nurses or clinical officers. Pre-cancer can also be removed by excision, often involving loop electrosurgical excision procedures (LEEPs): a local anesthetic is applied to the cervix and a hot wire is used to remove problematic cervical tissue. The use of LEEPs requires more training and expertise, but both ablations and LEEPs can be performed in clinics. Cone biopsies are performed with general anesthesia in an operating room. These procedures require more medical training and expertise than do ablations or LEEPs. Cone biopsies are 90 to 95 percent effective in getting rid of pre-cancer. In addition, patients who have had excisions, ablations, or cone biopsies can also be discharged the same day, making any one of these procedures a more practical option for women with cervical pre-cancer in countries or regions where price and lack of access present serious obstacles. G. F. Sawaya and K. Smith-McCune, "Cervical Cancer Screening," *Obstet Gynecol* **127**, no. 3 (Mar 2016): 459–67. https://doi.org/10.1097/AOG.0000000000001136 www.ncbi.nlm.nih.gov/pubmed/26855089

that care or unclear about the need for it. These deficiencies are usually at the heart of cancer prevention programs that don't succeed.

When No Means Yes: The Need for Top-Tier Testing

Even though Pap tests are highly reliable, on rare occasions, they fail. When a Pap smear result comes back negative, a woman can usually rest assured that she doesn't have abnormal cells on her cervix. But around 8 percent of the time, the Pap test comes back negative – even when disease is present. This is considered a "false negative" result.

The abnormalities leading to false negatives are usually found in the "endocervical canal" (between the outside of the cervix and the uterus) (Figure 5.3). The endocervical canal is harder to sample via Pap smear – making cancer harder to detect – especially in the part of the canal closest to the uterus. Studies have shown that Pap tests can miss up to 30 percent of endocervical canal abnormalities. Nonetheless, patients who regularly and repeatedly go for Pap smear testing are far more likely to get an accurate diagnosis, based on cervical cancer's growth and the law of averages.

Even though prevention is best for avoiding cervical cancer, Pap tests are less likely to pick up adenocarcinoma, a cancer that forms in the lining of the endocervix. Emma, a resident of New South Wales in Australia, developed adenocarcinoma after the diagnosis was missed on her Pap smear. When she received her diagnosis at twenty-nine, Emma also happened to be pregnant.

When I spoke with Emma in spring 2020, she recalled receiving her surprise diagnosis thirty-two weeks into her pregnancy while she was otherwise healthy and working as an elementary school teacher. Her previous five Pap smears had come back negative. But when she started having heavy vaginal bleeding, she was rushed to hospital, where doctors discovered a cancerous mass occupying part of her cervix.

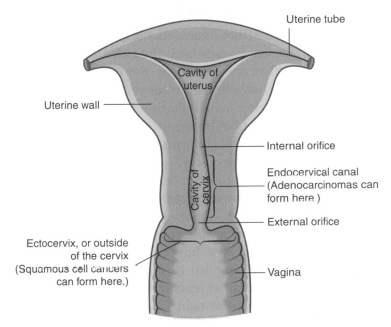

Figure 5.3 Cervical anatomy sites where cervical cancer forms
Source: Adapted from *Comprehensive Cervical Cancer Control: A Guide to Essential Practice.* WHO Guidelines Approved by the Guidelines Review Committee. Geneva, 2014.

Emma's treatment for cancer lasted a few months while she was caring for her newborn baby. Three and a half years later, she was free of the disease and planning for her second child via surrogacy with eggs she'd preserved before treatment. Just for peace of mind, she contacted the laboratory that evaluated her previous Pap smears to see if they had missed anything. "The tests still came back negative," she said. While Emma acknowledged the relative inability of Pap smears to detect her type of cancer, her experience hasn't changed her thinking about continuing to screen for cervical cancer.

Emma's key takeaway? *Keep going to the doctor regularly.* Emma takes all of the necessary precautions, knowing that timely medical checkups, including getting screened, are still the best way to prevent cervical cancer. The last thing she would want, she said, is to layer in additional obstacles to preventing cervical cancer. "I still tell everyone I know to get screened and get their tests."

The Power of Negative HPV-DNA

In the quest for even earlier, more reliable discovery of cervical abnormalities, physicians now have the HPV-DNA test, newer and more precise than the Pap smear. Not only will HPV-DNA testing detect the virus before it causes cellular abnormalities, it's better at detecting abnormalities in the endocervical canal.[6,7] Adding in HPV-DNA testing increases the rate of adenocarcinoma detection, and thereby protects patients like Emma from "slipping through the cracks."

In higher-income countries over the past twenty years, many of my colleagues and I have depended on the HPV-DNA test – in concert with the Pap smear – for detecting pre-cancer. The HPV-DNA test is the one I gave my patient Jennifer, allowing her to learn right away she had HPV, how common it was, and what sorts of risks having HPV implied. By the same token, HPV-DNA tests offer a powerful form of reassurance: when an HPV-DNA test is negative, there's a less than 1 percent chance that pre-cancer or cancer is present.[8] Excellent further research indicates that if both HPV-DNA and Pap tests are negative, the likelihood of cancer developing in the subsequent five years is less than one-tenth of 1 percent – good news indeed for women seeking to avoid cervical cancer.[9]

When it comes to offering successful cervical cancer screening programs, higher-income countries carry further advantages. Secondary prevention works not just because of reliable testing and follow-up treatment, but because most medical establishments have orderly monitoring systems. These systems provide recommended testing and treatment schedules for patients and track those who aren't keeping up with appointments. Tracking ensures women receive not only initial Pap tests but also all of the necessary follow-up care. Ultimately, women should receive an established system of checks and balances against cancer.

To be effective, screening for cervical cancer needs to be widespread and offered to all eligible women in the appropriate age group. Yet these monitoring systems are often absent or inefficient in countries without the political will or health care funds to make them a priority.

For regions of the world where Pap screening or HPV-DNA testing is neither affordable nor feasible, health care providers rely on simpler, less expensive screening tests. In African countries, and in India, for example, Visual Inspection with Acetic Acid (VIA) is the most common screening test for cervical cancer. VIA still involves an internal pelvic examination using a speculum. However, rather than using a Q-tip to collect a sample, acetic acid (vinegar-water) is applied to the cervix. After about a minute, abnormal areas of the cervix take on a whitish color. With training, a VIA provider can determine whether a whitish-looking abnormality requires treatment and provide that treatment on the spot, an approach called "Screen and Treat." And while it's less sophisticated and less reliable, VIA offers women in lower-income countries a modicum of protection against cervical cancer – protection that's better than no screening at all.

In lower-income regions with fewer clinics or providers, where patients may need to travel long or troublesome distances to medical clinics, the Screen and Treat method offers a pragmatic alternative. Typically requiring just one visit, Screen and Treat tests can save money and time for women who need to find childcare or leave work to see a health care provider, and fewer patients are lost to the follow-up process. What's more, nurses or clinical officers can be trained to perform VIA exams, helping to address the typical scarcity of skilled medical practitioners.

To perform VIA well, however, providers need significant training and ongoing supervision, and the treatment for cervical pre-cancer – usually ablation – needs to be made available. These additional expenses and requirements pose a heavy burden for countries without the funds or government support to supply them properly and consistently. So, despite their promise, few lower-income countries have established consistent, nationwide, affordable Screen and Treat programs.

Early Cancer Treatment Viable – but Expensive

While the HPV vaccine and cervical screening are effective ways to prevent cervical cancer, its incidence is more common in lower-income countries or marginalized communities within higher-income countries, where vaccination, screening, and follow-up treatment are often unavailable. When women get cervical cancer because they lack access to vaccines or screening – or in rarer cases, such as Emma's, *after* they've been screened – when they're diagnosed early, tertiary prevention measures can save their lives.

The success of tertiary prevention partly depends on cervical cancer's slow growth. Unlike other types of cancer, cervical cancer is less likely to spread via the lymph nodes or bloodstream, with the tumor usually confined to the cervix or adjacent tissue. Tertiary interventions usually involve treatment with surgery, radiation, chemotherapy, or a combination of all three, depending on tumor size and spread.

Unfortunately, women in lower-income countries usually have far fewer treatment options. Their governments are less likely to supply the necessary specialized equipment, facilities, and personnel. When persons with cervixes can access early treatment, the treatments themselves can lead to lifelong health problems or a diminished quality of life. Many would argue that it makes greater financial (and moral) sense to focus first on developing cheaper, more effective, and less invasive prevention programs. But until that happens, it's critical to be able to treat women with cervical cancer.

The Plight of Prevention Scarcity

In reality, the relative worldwide scarcity of the three prevention pillars goes a long way toward explaining the high death rate from cervical cancer. Given the barriers against fighting this disease in less affluent parts of the world, my initial apprehensions toward taking my first Pap test seem trite. At twenty-one, as I was about to tackle medical school, I was lucky enough to know how and why I needed to take those steps to avoid cervical cancer and to have them readily available to me.

When I began working in clinics in Liberia and Nicaragua, I encountered female patients whose country's minimal health care budgets limited their prevention options. As a doctor working in U.S. clinics, I came across women without medical insurance coverage who were struggling to take part in cervical cancer prevention regimens. What I would learn is that a seemingly preventable cancer continues to kill staggering numbers of women. Despite the sound science behind beating cervical cancer – through the body's own reset mechanism to clear HPV, as I explained to Jennifer, or the use of primary, secondary, and tertiary prevention combined with the cancer's slow growth, or even the effectiveness of health care monitoring systems for care and follow-up – this cancer is still winning out. As citizens of the world, we remain the losers.

6 THE TOLL
OF TREATMENT

Despite the outstanding promise of the human papillomavirus (HPV) vaccine and screening, every year more than 600,000 persons with cervixes around the world are stricken with cervical cancer. Without treatment, these people will die. Until we can achieve a sustained, worldwide effort toward preventing cervical cancer, we must rely on surgery, radiation, chemotherapy – and to a lesser degree, the newer approach of immunotherapy* – to prolong and sometimes save lives. In the short term, treatment for cervical cancer is a godsend. In this spirit, I celebrate the cancer-alleviating and curing measures we're able to offer those with cervical cancer, even while I call for a means to erase this cancer from the globe.

While effective cancer treatment is far better than no treatment at all, that treatment comes at a cost. Patients with access to surgery, radiation, and chemotherapy have a good chance of surviving this slow-growing cancer. But survival often equals long-term, life-altering consequences. Carol, a resident of northern California, knows these consequences all too well. She underwent all three of these types of treatment – and not just once. She survived, but her life has been irrevocably changed.

In 2011, Carol started bleeding after intercourse. As a forty-six-year-old single mom working full-time and raising two

---

* Immunotherapy is a less common type of cervical cancer treatment. It harnesses the power of the body's immune system to fight tumor cells. Immunotherapy is typically not used as a first-line therapy. L. Ferrall, K. Y. Lin, R. B. S. Roden, C. F. Hung, and T. C. Wu, "Cervical Cancer Immunotherapy: Facts and Hopes," *Clin Cancer Res* **27**, no. 18 (Sep 15 2021): 4953–73. https://doi.org/10.1158/1078-0432.CCR-20-2833 www.ncbi.nlm.nih.gov/pubmed/33888488

teenage sons, she found it challenging to schedule and attend a doctor's appointment, but she did so. The need to come in for her yearly pelvic examinations with the same provider, she said, had "been drummed into my head." Born too late to avail herself of the HPV vaccine, Carol took advantage of the best prevention available: regular Pap smear tests, which always came back normal. In 2008, at age forty-three, Carol received her first of the newer and more sophisticated HPV-DNA tests, which have since become more widely available. When those test results came back positive, Carol saw her provider twice at the recommended six-month intervals, each time receiving reassuring negative test results.

When she was bleeding in 2011, and an examination revealed a seven-centimeter mass on Carol's cervix, neither Carol nor her provider were prepared for the news. "It had literally been one year since my previous check. Everyone, including me, was so shocked." Because Carol's tumor was large, she needed two separate rounds of chemotherapy, a radical hysterectomy, and external radiation. While these treatments were lifesaving, each of them came at great sacrifice and without any promise of a cure.

Indeed, in 2012, Carol's cervical cancer came back, and she required a total pelvic exenteration surgery, one of the most complex and disfiguring surgeries a woman with reproductive cancer can undergo. An eleven- to twelve-hour surgery, pelvic exenteration is an invasive and grueling removal of all female reproductive organs, the bladder, and the rectum. In Carol's case, the lower half of her body was essentially "sewn shut," and she was left with bags on either side of her body for excreting waste.

"They felt it was the only option," Carol told me over Zoom one sunny September afternoon in 2020. Her easy smile conveyed warmth, but in her eyes, I saw a steely determination. "I decided to go for it," she said. Her recovery was prolonged. "Really, it took many months for my body to adjust," she said, "and for me to adjust to having these bags, and to get my energy back."

I asked Carol to describe how she'd adjusted to losing her bladder and rectum, marveling at her upbeat attitude. "Well, I have to use some humor to help me deal with it," she replied. Carol calls her urostomy, the new opening that allows her urine to be directed away from her bladder and into a collection bag, "Fred." Her colostomy, the opening created to catch her stool in a separate collection bag, is "Ethel."

"I can be in a meeting for work, and all of a sudden Ethel will start making these noises," Carol said. "The fun part is no one can tell where the noise is coming from. Ethel and I get to share the secret," she added, with a mischievous smile. Carol admitted that it took her at least a year to be able to laugh about her circumstances. "A very long, difficult year," she said. "But where would I be without Fred and Ethel?"

Carol's exenteration didn't offer her the cure she'd hoped for – or even much breathing room – before her cancer recurred in 2013. She was treated with chemotherapy and, "too soon after that," had another recurrence in 2015, for which she received immunotherapy. In 2016, the cancer came back a fourth time, requiring further chemotherapy.

Carol's treatments have kept her cancer at bay, but each one has taken its toll. Carol said she still gets terrible "scanxiety" before each semiannual follow-up PET scan or CT scan, a familiar complaint from many cervical cancer survivors and a reminder that cervical cancer treatment is really only the beginning of a lifelong relationship with this disease. Survivorship is often marked by the ongoing trauma of anxiety and fear of recurrence: "How long before I will hear the results of the test?" "Will my CT scan show anything?" "Is my cancer back?"

In addition to Carol's physical and emotional trials, she's also had to come to terms with a kind of physical disfigurement few women contemplate. "I now have a Barbie Butt," she told me matter-of-factly. "I have a clitoris, but no vagina and no rectum. It is just all sewed-up and shiny there – just like Barbie." I've witnessed the wide range of treatments associated with cervical cancer, but still find it difficult to process what Carol endured and continues to endure. Her treatments saved her life but ravaged her body.

> *"I now have a Barbie Butt," she told me matter-of-factly.*

Cervical Cancer Treatment: The Humbling Truth

Not every person with cervical cancer will endure the long, complex treatment Carol went through. Carol's pelvic exenteration surgery was a very rare form of cervical cancer treatment. When cancer is caught early enough, and treatment takes place soon thereafter, persons with cervixes can go on to live relatively normal lives. Even Carol, despite her difficult surgery, has found a way to get on with her life through her courage and sense of humor. But every form of treatment exacts a toll, and the size of that toll depends on many factors, including access to these treatments as soon as possible after diagnosis.

Treatment for cervical cancer is determined by the size and spread of the tumor, indicated by stages (Figure 6.1). Stages 1 through 4 refer to the spread of cancer, and an A or B designates its size. Stage 1 cervical cancer means that cancer is confined to the cervix, for example, while Stage 1A points to a half-centimeter, microscopic tumor, and Stage 1B describes a larger-than-half-centimeter tumor within the cervix. Stage 2 means the cancer has grown beyond the cervix and uterus but hasn't spread to the pelvic walls or lower part of the vagina. Once the cancer has spread to these areas, it's considered Stage 3, and may be blocking the ureters. Stage 4 cervical cancer has grown into the bladder or rectum or spread to organs like the lungs or bones. At any stage, cancer is harder to cure once it has spread to the lymph nodes. And, when cervical cancer reaches Stage 3 or 4, the tumor has spread beyond the cervix, requiring much more extensive treatment. Unsurprisingly, as the cancer spreads to other parts of the body, surviving cervical cancer at this stage becomes increasingly unlikely.

Cervical cancer Stage 1B (76–92%)

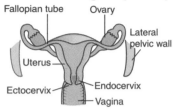

Cervical cancer Stage 2A (73–90%)

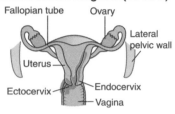

Cervical cancer Stage 2B (60–84%)

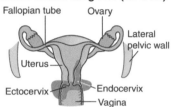

Cervical cancer Stage 3A (40–50%)

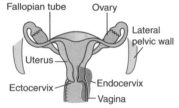

Cervical cancer Stage 3B (37–42%)

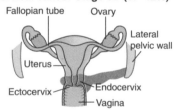

Cervical cancer Stage 4A (18–32%)

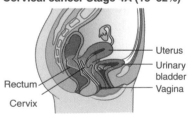

Cervical cancer Stage 4B (13–24%)

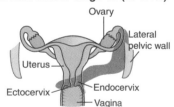

Figure 6.1 Cross-section illustrations of a cervix showing cervical cancer stages and survival rates

Source: "What Is the Survival Rate of Patients with Cervical Cancer at Different Stages?" https://mediglobus.com/what-is-the-survival-rate-of-patients-with-cervical-cancer-at-different-stages/. Accessed Jan 27, 2023.

An early diagnosis can save a life but grant a life-altering burden. In the vast majority of cases, even with surgery-only treatment, women usually require hysterectomies and thereby lose their ability to bear children. In only the most minor Stage 1A cases of cervical cancer, a patient might be able to keep her uterus while still having part or all of her cervix removed. In other words, even "good surgical outcomes" can mean long-term sacrifice – along with long-term angst and heartbreak.

A Life Saved but Forever Altered

Surgically treating Stage IB and smaller Stage 2A cervical cancer almost always requires what is aptly called a "radical" hysterectomy: removal of the uterus, cervix, and a portion of the vagina (Figure 6.2). A surgeon will also excise extra tissue around the cervix to reduce the likelihood of a recurrence and remove

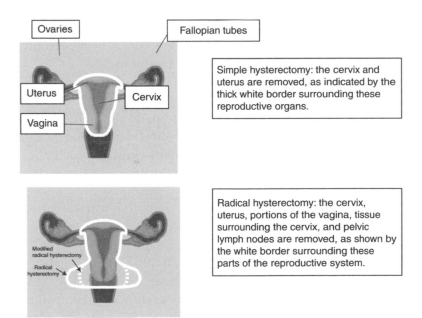

Figure 6.2 Cross-section illustrations of a cervix showing surgical hysterectomy margins
Source: Adapted from *Comprehensive Cervical Cancer Control: A Guide to Essential Practice*. WHO Guidelines Approved by the Guidelines Review Committee, 182. Geneva, 2014.

pelvic lymph nodes to test for further cancer spread. This is hardly a simple operation. Radical hysterectomies are performed by obstetrician gynecologists – often gynecologic oncologists – who've received years of additional training because of the risks associated with operating in proximity to large blood vessels and nerves lying in the pelvis or along the aorta adjacent to the lymph nodes. Recovery involves four to six days in hospital, and typically six to eight weeks more at home, a burden for any person of means, but an extra challenge for the uninsured or for those upon whom children, elders, neighbors, partners, jobs, and communities depend.

For many women with cervical cancer, even a radical hysterectomy isn't an option. If the tumor is larger than four to five centimeters, gynecologic oncologists will usually order radiation. If the cancer has spread outside the cervix, then radiation is also required, regardless of the size of the initial cervical tumor. Despite receiving regular screening, Carol developed a seven-centimeter tumor. (Like Emma, Carol had adenocarcinoma.) Before becoming a candidate for a radical hysterectomy, Carol first needed radiation to shrink the tumor.

Radiation is a common and proven treatment option. It kills cancer cells by damaging their DNA and thereby inhibiting their growth. Radiation can be applied externally through external beams (a machine outside the body directs radiation beams toward specific cancer sites) or internally through brachytherapy (the source of radiation is put into the vagina or tissue close to the cervix), or both.

As with radical hysterectomies, radiation often batters a woman's body and comes with painful and even permanent aftereffects. After weeks of external beam radiation, women often experience bowel pain and cramping, fecal urgency – the constant feeling of needing to have a bowel movement, even if stool is not present – diarrhea, difficulty controlling urine and bladder urges, and generalized pain. In some women, the side effects of external radiation are immediate, and they only resolve later on, after treatment. Carol, for instance, described herself as "so fortunate," because her radiation side effects lasted no longer than her treatment.

For other women, however, diarrhea, nausea, vomiting, and stomach cramps – referred to as "radiation enteritis" – may start a few weeks or even a few months after the full course of radiation. Radiation enteritis can sometimes linger for years. Its sufferers might find their gratitude for a possible cure cruelly tempered by the pain, frustration, and loneliness accompanying the misery of a malfunctioning bowel.

Emily, a resident of Iowa diagnosed at thirty with Stage 2B cervical cancer, faced complications following both internal and external radiation treatment. "You are young, and you will do well," her care team had told her. The team may have been well meaning, but to Emily, their words were painfully inaccurate. The idea of Emily's youth giving her the edge failed to account for her body's devastating reaction to radiation – the chronic side effects, she said, that dwarfed and changed her life forever.

Three months after radiation treatment, Emily developed a debilitating form of radiation enteritis. Almost daily, she experienced severe cramping, accompanied by multiple bouts of diarrhea. For four years, she experienced such severe intestinal pain and cramps that she "could not stand or walk when they hit. I just had to go to bed until they would lessen."

Emily reached out repeatedly for medical care to relieve her symptoms, but found no one with sufficient experience or knowledge of her condition. For four years, she was reduced to a diet consisting largely of pureed baby food, forced to give up her career as a scientific field researcher because she could no longer perform her field duties. She also ended her relationship with her fiancé because, in spite of his support, she felt her poor health precluded her from being in a relationship. "I was so overwhelmed with how awful I felt," she said.

Like so many cervical cancer patients, Emily grew increasingly isolated. "I was thirty-one and I lost all my social life, because I would cancel plans at the last minute if the cramps hit hard. I could never eat the food at people's houses or a restaurant, so people quit inviting me, and if I did go to a restaurant, I could never be far from a bathroom." Finally, in the fourth year after her diagnosis, and after her fourth trip to an emergency room for debilitating intestinal pain, an ER doctor suggested hyperbaric oxygen treatments,* and Emily started to get some relief. "Now, instead of missing work one to two times a week due to cramps, it has become once a month or every other month."

"Cancer does not end with treatment," Emily pointed out. "It's a lifelong thing." Emily was echoing a truth I'd heard from Nina, after her thirty-eight-year-old daughter died of cervical cancer. "Just because I *look* okay does not mean I *am* okay," Teolita once told her mother. "It is a confusing reality to have a 'normal' physical appearance while I watch my life be devastated by all these changes."

"It is a confusing reality to have a 'normal' physical appearance while I watch my life be devastated by all these changes."

Emily and Teolita's experiences reflect the fact that treatment may or may not save a life – Emily survived; Teolita didn't – but treatment always takes something from the person fighting for theirs.

While Emily's suffering arose from external beam treatment, brachytherapy can bring equally brutal outcomes. Despite receiving sedatives for these procedures, several women I interviewed described an excruciatingly painful and traumatic encounter with brachytherapy treatment – one they recall instantly, many years after the fact.

The type of instrument used for brachytherapy depends on where the cancer has spread (Figure 6.3). If cancer is just in the cervix, intrauterine tandems and vaginal cylinders are inserted

---

* Hyperbaric oxygen treatment involves breathing pure oxygen in a pressurized environment to markedly increase the oxygen level in the bloodstream. This form of treatment can promote tissue healing by boosting oxygen levels in tissue damaged by radiation. P. Craighead, M. A. Shea-Budgell, J. Nation, *et al.*, "Hyperbaric Oxygen Therapy for Late Radiation Tissue Injury in Gynecologic Malignancies," *Curr Oncol* **18**, no. 5 (Oct 2011): 220–7. https://doi.org/10.3747/co.v18i5.767 www.ncbi.nlm.nih.gov/pubmed/21980249

(a)

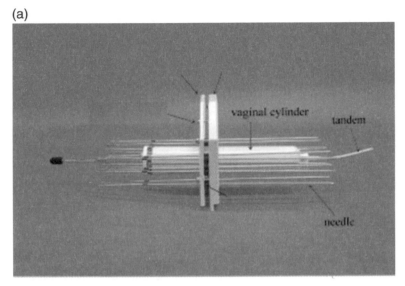

(b)

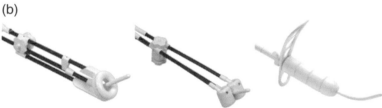

Figure 6.3 Examples of brachytherapy devices placed in the vagina to treat cervical cancer. (a) Syed needle interstitial brachytherapy device.
Source: Reused with permission from Nose T, Onoe T, Otani Y, Oguchi M, Yamashita T. A simple technique to minimize needle displacement in gynecologic interstitial brachytherapy: Use of fully stretched elastic tapes. Brachytherapy. 2016 May-Jun;15(3):347-352. doi: 10.1016/j. brachy.2016.02.009. Epub 2016 Mar 28. PMID: 27032994
(b) Tandem and ovoids, and vaginal cylinder brachytherapy devices.
Source: Hasan, Y., Song, W.Y., Fisher, C. (2019). Intracavitary Brachytherapy: Definitive, Preoperative, and Adjuvant (Cervix, Uterine, and Vaginal). In: Albuquerque, K., Beriwal, S., Viswanathan, A., Erickson, B. (eds) Radiation Therapy Techniques for Gynecological Cancers. Practical Guides in Radiation Oncology. Springer, Cham. https://doi.org/10.1007/978-3-030-01443-8_8

directly into the cervix and vagina. If the cancer has spread beyond the cervix and into the vagina and paracervical tissue, an effective but draconian-looking instrument known as a "Syed-type interstitial implant" may be inserted into the vagina. The needles on this device contain radioactive material that pummels the tumor while a cylinder holds the apparatus in place. Syed radiation treatment increases the radiation dose to the paracervical tissue.

Compared with external radiation, Syed treatment may be more effective in reducing or eliminating a tumor spreading outside the cervix.[1] Syed treatment can also cause fewer bladder, bowel, and intestinal function side effects. However, sedation alone does little to help patients withstand the pain of implanting Syed needles; patients typically require general anesthesia.

Before her debilitating external beam therapy and subsequent radiation enteritis, *devastating* was the word Emily used to describe brachytherapy treatment "I just laid there, unable to move, unable to wipe my tears – and cried the whole time. I had no idea how awful it was going to be." Other cervical cancer survivors described not only their struggles with grueling treatment, but also the shocking reality of post-radiation life. As Emily put it: "I was told I would lose my fertility. At thirty years old, that was hard enough. But to pile on all the other trauma and side effects made the first four years after my treatment a huge, day-to-day struggle.

"Survivorship," she added: "it's a big deal."

"I was told I would lose my fertility. At thirty years old, that was hard enough. But to pile on all the other trauma and side effects made the first four years after my treatment a huge, day-to-day struggle.

"Survivorship," she added: "it's a big deal."

Radiation might have saved Emily's life, and has certainly spared the lives of countless other women, and not all women experience rare, but life-changing, post-treatment side effects.[2] What unites these women, however, is the dramatic effect of brachytherapy on the vagina. All of the brachytherapy patients I spoke with told me stories of vaginal narrowing, scarring, discomfort, or pain from sexual penetration, and bleeding after intercourse – all of which had devastating effects on their sexuality. Some of the women I interviewed told me they were eventually able to have intercourse, but many whom I spoke with were not.

Chemoradiation: Effective but Brutal

For women diagnosed with cervical cancer beyond Stage 1A, or for those managing recurrences, the standard of care may combine treatment options: surgery, chemotherapy, and radiation, with chemotherapy and radiation (chemoradiation) typically offered at the same time. When Carol's lymph nodes were removed and found positive for cancer, she needed chemoradiation. And while chemoradiation – available since the 1950s – improves the chances of survival, its consequent side effects are even more unpleasant than radiation alone, often including increased nausea and vomiting, or nerve pain and tingling in the feet.

But for the majority of women undergoing cervical cancer treatment, the most devastating loss is the subsequent inability to bear a child. Patients with tumors small enough to require removal or partial removal of the cervix may retain some chance of childbearing, but for most, infertility is a given. Even if a woman's treatment doesn't require a hysterectomy, radiation treatment can destroy fertility by damaging the uterus, and chemoradiation can damage the eggs in the ovaries or prompt early menopause. In addition to the fear, loneliness, anxiety, pain, sexual dysfunction, and lifelong, body-altering complications caused by these cancer treatments, in order to save her own life, a woman must exchange her ability to create a new one. It's hard to imagine a crueler trade.

The Dollars-and-Cents Cost of Treatment

In addition to the soul-crushing costs of cervical cancer that have nothing to do with money, cervical cancer sufferers must also face the steep price tag of treatment. In 2016, Canadian researchers evaluated the cost of treatment for 779 women diagnosed with cervical cancer at around age forty-nine. Their findings: the mean costs in the first year after diagnosis amounted to more than $31,000 USD. For those who died within that year – likely diagnosed at a more advanced stage – the price was more than $54,500 USD. In-patient hospitalizations and cancer-related care were the two biggest costs.

In England in 2014, the National Health Service (NHS) published findings on the average NHS cost per person diagnosed with Stage 2 or later cervical cancer at more than £19,000 (in excess of $26,000 USD).[3] In looking at overall treatment costs in the United States, a study found that between 2010 and 2020, the nation spent $1.6 billion USD a year treating cervical cancer. As we'll see, these numbers don't begin to account for the cost of lost productivity among working women or the almost incalculable loss of unpaid labor women provide in caring for children, homes, neighbors, elders, and communities.

Keep in mind that this data only addresses treatment costs in higher-income countries, where such treatment is accessible. Imagine how different Carol's and Emily's stories would be if they were from Madagascar and Cambodia, instead of California and Iowa. As we will explore in the next chapters, hundreds of thousands of persons with cervixes around the world aren't even "lucky enough" to be offered treatment for their cervical cancer. In some cases, these cancer sufferers cannot personally afford treatment or it's simply unavailable. There's no nice way to say it: for many women around the world, a diagnosis of cervical cancer is a death sentence.

This is what makes primary and secondary prevention – vaccination and screening – so critical to sparing women cervical cancer. For the hundreds of thousands of women in lower-income countries with zero hope of accessing treatment, no matter the pain, no matter the emotional and physical cost they might be willing to pay in return for their lives, vaccination and screening are not just the most cost-effective options. They are the *only* options.

Carol and Emily would agree. I am humbled by their resilience, courage, and power. They are robust in grabbing each day, fiercely living sunrise to sunset, perhaps as only someone can after facing four cervical cancer recurrences or four years of radiation enteritis. They've both expressed to me how deeply grateful they were to access lifesaving medical care. But I know they would gladly trade their newfound wisdom to have avoided these difficult treatments altogether.

Carol and Emily are strong advocates for vaccination and screening, and while I celebrate the incredible treatments that save lives, I wholeheartedly join them in their call. We must achieve a sustained, worldwide effort toward preventing cervical cancer. I'm thankful for treatment for cervical cancer – and unequivocal that it be provided to those who need it, when they need it. But vaccination and screening remain the key to ending this disease for good.

7 GASOLINE ON THE FIRE: WHEN HIV MEETS HPV

I'm grateful for the remarkable tools we already have to combat cervical cancer. When I consider the effectiveness of vaccination and screening, and the sophistication of surgery, chemotherapy, and radiation, the call to eliminate this cancer becomes more than just wishful thinking: it engenders hope. I wholeheartedly believe that when all 194 member countries of the World Health Organization pledged to join this fight in 2020, they signed on to a realistic goal.

At the same time, a particular and deadly threat lies in wait for many of these countries. That threat is largely concentrated in Africa, but it's one we need to address together. I'm referring to another sexually transmitted virus familiar to all of us: the human immunodeficiency virus, or HIV.

Identified in the 1980s, HIV terrorized the world for years until scientists created antiretroviral treatments, and HIV became a chronic, but livable, condition. While antiretrovirals were initially only available in higher-income countries, they've now made life longer and more manageable for persons with this debilitating viral infection in lower-income countries. Still, HIV ravages the globe. At the end of 2020, nearly 40 million people were living with HIV, over two-thirds of them in Africa.[1] Every week, roughly 5,000 young women aged fifteen to twenty-four become infected with HIV, and in sub-Saharan Africa, six in seven new HIV infections occur among fifteen- to nineteen-year-old girls.[2] In the lower-income world, where access to HIV treatment and even prevention face tremendous financial, logistical, and social obstacles, HIV remains a very real terror: killing more than 600,000 people every year.

Now, let's imagine adding a common HPV infection to a patient already infected with HIV, and it's like tossing gasoline on a fire. A woman with HIV is six times more likely to die of cervical cancer than a woman without HIV.[3] Six times! Together, HIV and HPV form a lethal, seemingly unstoppable, force.

HIV: A Cervical Cancer Accelerant

Human immunodeficiency virus compromises the body's immune responses, and that's not good news in combating the virus causing cervical cancer. Remember, 80 percent of sexually active people will contract one or more HPV infections in their lifetime, but the body's immune system usually takes care of that, preventing the virus from persisting long enough to cause cancer. A woman with a healthy immune system may resolve an HPV infection within a few months. But with an HIV-compromised immune system, the body struggles to clear the virus,[4,5] and HPV may linger in the cervix for as long as twelve to eighteen months.[6] This longer "lingering time" gives high-risk types of HPV more time to do damage: effecting the kind of change in cervical cells that leads to pre-cancer.

Typically, it takes ten to twenty years for an HPV infection to result in cancer – what medicine calls "the latency period." But in an HIV-compromised immune system, cancer can develop as quickly as three to five years. This holds significant implications for the success of cervical cancer screening programs, which rely on a longer latency period. Women without HIV are advised to get Pap smear screening once every three years, while women living with HIV are told to get Pap screening every year until they receive a few years of normal test results. But for a person with a cervix infected with HIV and a high-risk HPV type, pre-cancer can morph into cancer faster than screening can pick it up.

HIV mixed with HPV: lethal, indeed.

Human immunodeficiency virus also makes cervical cancer harder to treat. The success rate for ablation – which destroys precancerous cells from the cervix – ranges from 85 to 90 percent in women without an HIV infection. But among women infected with HIV, some studies found that the rate of success for ablation treatment plummeted to between 40 and 60 percent.[7] Women with HIV may have better success with excision treatment, or LEEPs (loop electrosurgical excision procedures, described in Chapter 5), which, in some studies, were up to 95 percent effective in preventing cancer.

Excision therapy, however, requires more expensive equipment and better trained providers, it carries an increased risk of post-procedure complications, and it requires more post-procedural visits. And, unlike ablation, which can often be done in a local clinic, excision adds to patient burden: it's generally performed in large, urban clinics or in hospitals, adding longer possible waiting times, extra costs, and the complications of travel. For women in lower-income countries or underresourced regions, excision treatment is often out of reach. As women struggle to make appointments, arrange travel and childcare, gather the money necessary for treatment, travel, and lost work time, they are delaying treatment, allowing time for pre-cancer to develop into cancer.

Keep in mind that these challenges remain the "privilege" of women living in countries that offer excision therapy at all. Despite studies that cite excision as the cervical pre-cancer treatment of choice for women living with HIV, access to excision treatment is either limited or unavailable in lower-income countries, the very same countries with the highest rates of HIV. When I was working in Namibia in 2017, only a few locations in the country could provide LEEP; while I was in Malawi in 2018, women had to travel to major cities for LEEP treatment. This lack of access to LEEP makes ablation therapy more readily available for women with both pre-cancer and HIV, yet less effective in preventing pre-cancer from becoming cancer.

The Center of the Global Inferno

Human immunodeficiency virus infection continues to plague southern and eastern Africa. It should be no surprise that cervical cancer rates are soaring there as well. Africa – the global epicenter of both HIV and cervical cancer incidence and death – remains the core of the HIV–HPV (human papillomavirus) inferno.

In 2020, an international group of cancer epidemiologists and HIV researchers published findings in *Lancet Global Health* showing that almost 6 percent of new global cervical cancer cases – around 33,000 every year – were diagnosed in women living with HIV, despite a less than 1 percent global prevalence of HIV (Figure 7.1).[3] This same study identified southern and eastern Africa as regions most affected by combined HIV–HPV infections.[8] It revealed that almost two-thirds (around 64 percent) of female cervical cancer sufferers in southern Africa were also living with HIV. More than 27 percent of women in eastern Africa struggled with the same deadly disease duo.[9]

Social and Cultural Norms Set the "HIV Fire" Ablaze

Child marriage – what the United Nations calls "any formal marriage or informal union between a child under eighteen and an adult or another child" – remains a common practice in many parts of the world. Generally, child marriage takes place in lower-income countries, and in particular, within the HIV–HPV-burdened regions of southern and eastern Africa (Figure 7.2). In fact, 20 to 30 percent of child marriages in these regions involve girls younger than fifteen.[10] This practice denies girls the right to choose their sexual partners, and the striking power imbalance between man and child often leaves these young wives with no say in their partner's sexual behaviors, putting them at dire risk of contracting fast-spreading HIV and HPV.

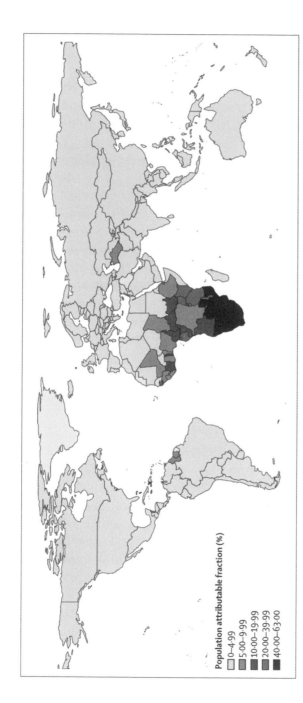

Figure 7.1 Population percentages of cervical cancer sufferers with HIV

Source: Stelzle, D., L. F. Tanaka, K. K. Lee, et al. "Estimates of the Global Burden of Cervical Cancer Associated with HIV." *Lancet Glob Health* **9**, no. 2 (Feb 2021): e161–e69.

Population attributable fraction (%)

- 0–4·99
- 5·00–9·99
- 10·00–19·99
- 20·00–39·99
- 40·00–63·00

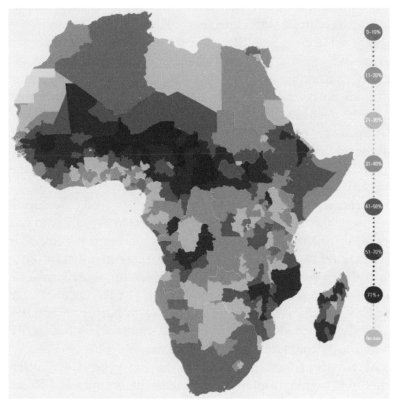

Figure 7.2 Prevalence of child brides in African countries
Source: https://data.unicef.org/resources/harmful-practices-in-africa/.
Accessed April 14, 2023.

During my decades of working with women across the world, I have met many women subjected to the practice of child marriage, and I've seen typical medical outcomes of socially sanctioned relationships where equal power and consent do not exist. Allow me to tell you the story of Florence.

Florence lived in a small village in central Guinea on the west coast of Africa. The fifth child of her family, Florence longed to go to school but was never given the option. Educating sons was the family's priority, while Florence and her sisters stayed home to help out on their small family farm, fetching water to feed the animals and working alongside their mother to harvest cashews. Florence knew her future was to be a wife and mother, and perhaps run a small business, such as a roadside stand.

When Florence was fifteen, a man offered her father two goats and a year's food provisions in exchange for marriage, and her father agreed. Despite being anxious about marrying a much older man she didn't know, Florence accepted her father's decision. In accordance with village expectations, Florence was pregnant after being married for a few months. The local primary health care clinic offered prenatal care services. During her first-ever prenatal visit, Florence learned she was HIV-positive. She was sixteen.

Florence was lucky enough to receive HIV medicine during her pregnancy to prevent HIV transmission to her son, who was born healthy and HIV-free. She was also lucky to have regular HIV care for the next nine years. Every three months, Florence dutifully traveled to the HIV clinic to pick up her HIV medication. By now, she was a mother of four. But Florence's village didn't offer the HPV vaccine to girls or to boys, and her HIV clinic did not conduct routine cervical cancer screening on HIV patients, putting Florence at terrible risk.

At twenty-six, Florence started having yellowish, "rotten smelling" vaginal discharge that occasionally contained blood. She began developing lower back pain. She told the HIV clinic provider, who conducted a pelvic exam and discovered a large, hard, irregular mass at the top of her vagina that bled to the touch. Florence had advanced cervical cancer. She died nine months later, at twenty-seven, leaving behind four children age ten and under.

Florence's HIV infection ramped up the progression of her HPV infection to cancer. When HIV isn't present, women typically develop cervical cancer at around forty-five. Florence was barely half that age. As a married teenager, Florence was in no position to understand or advocate for her sexual health. She lacked the power to insist on monogamy or disease prevention. Socially sanctioned by her culture and her own family, Florence's child marriage put her at especially high risk. Her outcome was tragic – but not unusual.

Child marriage represents a fearsome accelerant thrown on the fire of cervical cancer raging across parts of Africa. While the practice can't be linked directly to HIV and cervical cancer, its common features – early sexual onset and frequent unsafe sex – *can* be directly linked to higher rates of HIV and HPV. A 2019 study examined systemic factors underlying child marriage and HIV acquisition. These common factors include "structural inequalities that drive girls' vulnerability: early sexual onset, unsafe sex, frequency of sex, age-disparate relationships, low educational attainment, limited access to information and services, social isolation, and experience of intimate partner violence."[11]

The lack of power, information, and social support for child brides must surely affect their ability to know about or access cancer prevention and treatment measures. At fifteen, Florence was powerless to refuse marriage. She lacked the power to ask her future husband to get an HIV test or use condoms. Countries that still condone the "giving away" of teenage girls – young women who can't insist or even ask that their partners use condoms, get an HIV test, or disclose their HIV status – dramatically diminish efforts to stop HIV, and thereby, cervical cancer.

Sexual Stigma and Double Standards

When a woman in a southern or eastern African country carries both HPV and HIV, she staggers under the weight of stigma. And in cultures with sexual double standards for men and women and deep-rooted stigma around women's sexuality, that shame seems to fall disproportionately on women. Unfortunately, the stigma associated with sexually transmitted infection represents a key barrier to preventing and treating it.

In my three decades of providing medical care to women at a public hospital with patients from all over the globe, I remain amazed that a woman will be found "at fault" and stigmatized when it comes to sexually transmitted infections, while a man rarely is subjected to the same social consequences. The shame associated with a disease acquired by sex seems to be solely borne by females.

In the same regions that practice child marriage and hold women to harsh sexual standards, men are also known to practice polygamy, or multiple marriages, exponentially raising a women's likelihood of contracting HIV and HPV. When a woman is having sex with someone who's had multiple partners, and she's unprotected by vaccination or condom use, she is also exponentially exposed.

There is an established link between risky sexual behaviors or multiple partners and the danger of acquiring HIV. While working as a gynecologist overseas, I've seen many women become HIV-positive after only having one sexual partner. While no woman deserves the pain of social stigma, the automatic branding of an HIV-positive person as someone who engages in risky sexual behaviors seems deeply unfair. A child bride often never has intercourse before marriage. Her husband gives her HIV. Her husband gives her HPV. Her husband gets her pregnant. Women in these cultures, especially child brides, are put at risk and then made to bear the stigma, along with the health consequences, of that risk.

In addition to the perils of child marriage and sexual stigma, pregnancy poses a risk in acquiring HIV and, therefore, cervical cancer. Pregnancy alters the immunology and anatomy of cervical cells, and breastfeeding causes further hormonal and physical changes in the cervix. These changes leave women more susceptible to contracting HIV while they're pregnant or during the first six months after delivery.[12] In countries where closely spaced pregnancies are the norm, pregnancy becomes another high-risk component for HIV, HPV, and cervical cancer. The southern and eastern African countries bearing the highest rates of HIV also experience some of the highest birth rates in the world.[13]

Studies undertaken as early as 2011 of women from seven sub-Saharan African countries showed pregnant women were twice as likely to be infected by a partner's HIV as women who weren't pregnant. A subsequent study conducted in 2018 in the same region found a rate among women prior to pregnancy of 1 HIV acquisition per 1,000 exposures of intercourse or other sexual activity. But women pregnant at fourteen weeks or more were three times more likely to acquire HIV per exposure, and for the first six months after delivery, breastfeeding women were four times more likely to become HIV-positive.[14]

Many women, like Florence, in lower-income countries only learn of their HIV-positive status during their first pregnancies. For women in regions with minimal health care resources, pregnancy is often their first interaction with a health care provider. Ironically, then, while pregnancy is a risk factor for acquiring HIV, it's also a time when women can test and receive care for HIV, providing it's available. When Florence learned she was HIV-positive during her first pregnancy, she received regular HIV care and could use antiretroviral medicines to prevent mother–baby HIV transmission. What Florence was not afforded, however, was the opportunity to know her HPV status.

Taking Advantage of the Lethal HIV–HPV Link

Improvements in HIV research and the reduced cost of HIV medications have increased the life spans of women living with HIV. But these advancements bear a shadow side: women who would have previously died swiftly of HIV are now more vulnerable to other diseases, such as cervical cancer.

As the world began advocating for greater care for HIV-positive people, they missed a tremendous opportunity to link that care to other needs. HIV-positive women require a particular screening regimen that factors in HIV's accelerant effect on HPV, making HPV more likely to develop into cervical cancer. When HPV care is linked to HIV care, it offers women with HIV a chance to extinguish that additional threat.

In higher-income countries, the message to screen frequently for cervical cancer is well publicized among women with HIV whose cervical immune systems remain permanently compromised, despite regular HIV treatment. These women are often part of a centralized clinical tracking system to reduce their cervical cancer risks. Yet, in lower-income countries like Africa in particular, it's still uncommon for HIV-positive women to receive specialized screening against cervical cancer.

As part of their advocacy for cervical cancer care, the World Health Organization and funding agencies such as PEPFAR (the U.S. President's Emergency Plan for AIDS Relief) have begun to account for the prevalence of HPV in HIV-positive patients, with particular implications for high-HIV populations in lower-income African countries. Combating increased cervical cancer in women with HIV has led to a push for earlier and more frequent cervical cancer screening appointments.* The WHO recommends that cervical cancer screenings for women living with HIV begin at twenty-five (as opposed to thirty for women without HIV) and include screening tests and treatment designed for compromised immune systems. In 2018, PEPFAR announced a "Go Further" campaign to link cervical cancer screening with established HIV interventions.[15] A growing number of clinics in Africa have started offering dual services for screening and treating HIV and cervical cancer – accounting for the extra rigor required to keep cervical cancer at bay.

But questions remain over the degree to which the medical community can leverage the connection between HIV and cervical cancer. Global science has yet to untangle the precise physiological interplay between HPV and HIV. We can screen and treat pre-cancer more often and earlier in HIV-positive patients, but we cannot eliminate HIV's intensifying impact on HPV. Even when HIV treatment restores a woman's HIV-infected immune system, aggressive growth of HPV pre-cancer and cervical cancer can persist. Scientists are querying the perplexing persistence of HPV even when HIV has been controlled. Some posit that HIV

---

* Cervical cancer does not decrease to the same degree as other cancers associated with diminished immune function. For instance, Kaposi's sarcoma and lymphoma strike individuals with depleted immune activity and AIDS, but once their immune function is restored, these cancers abate. The same cannot be said for cervical cancer, which does not return to the HIV-negative degree of disease, even when antiretroviral therapy restores immune function. P. E. Castle, M. H. Einstein, and V. V. Sahasrabuddhe, "Cervical Cancer Prevention and Control in Women Living with Human Immunodeficiency Virus," *CA Cancer J Clin* **71**, no. 6 (Nov 2021): 505–26. https://doi.org/10.3322/caac.21696. www .ncbi.nlm.nih.gov/pubmed/34499351

medications – while powerful in restoring the immune system – are stymied by the possibility of HPV permanently altering the genetic code of cervical cells.[16,17] Until science better understands HIV's effect on HPV, the best we can do is screen and treat pre-cancer in HIV-positive women as frequently as recommended. Lower-income countries in particular will need to develop medical services that consider the compromised immune systems of women living with HIV. To provide these services, they will likely require the financial support of higher-income countries.

Extinguishing the Inferno

Given the combustible nature of HPV in a body already infected with HIV, slowing the rate of HIV becomes instrumental in stopping cervical cancer. Without a commitment to stopping HIV spread, cervical cancer will remain exceedingly difficult to eliminate in HIV-beleaguered countries.

Fighting the fiery mix of HIV and HPV requires a willingness to examine underlying inequalities between the sexes, and varying gender roles and expectations between countries and regions. The story of HIV in women is often a story of lack of empowerment, just as cervical cancer is a marker of inequity. As long as society allows women like Florence to remain subservient to men, women remain vulnerable to diseases like HIV and cervical cancer.

By elevating these women and their ability to negotiate important conversations with their partners, we empower them to make their own decisions about their health. When women are empowered to advocate for their health, make their own choices for marriage, have a say in family size and planning, and find financial sustainability outside of their roles as wives or mothers, they will be in a position to address the spread of HIV that threatens them, their sisters, their daughters, and their fellow citizens. Successful efforts to extinguish the inferno of HIV–HPV deaths require the participation of everyone, including the women who are at greatest risk of being burned.

Part Three
The Prevention Problem

8 THE DEADLY LINK BETWEEN INEQUALITY AND CERVICAL CANCER

In 2011, Kim, an American working mother of eight children, started making regular trips to Haiti as part of a volunteer church group based in Cincinnati, Ohio. It was during one of these trips that Kim met Elvia. Their cross-cultural friendship would span their differences. It would carry life-affirming – as well as life-altering – implications.

When the two women met, Elvia was working as a street vendor to help support her two young children. She sold drinks and snacks in front of her home in Port-au-Prince, the town where Kim's volunteer group taught technology skills to Haitian children, and the neighborhood where Kim often stayed. Elvia's and Kim's children often played together, roaming effortlessly between the two households. Kim and Elvia grew just as comfortable with each other. During Kim's visits back and forth from the United States, the two friends remained in close contact.

On one of those ordinary days when Kim and Elvia were enjoying time together in Port-au-Prince, a neighbor offered to snap a photo of Kim, Elvia, and Elvia's children just outside their neighbor's home (Figure 8.1). Kim now finds it chilling to look at the photograph she keeps nearby: on that very day, both of them unknowingly had cervical tumors growing inside them. And while Kim and Elvia shared the same type of cancer, they were instantly separated by vast differences in accessing cervical cancer treatment.

When she returned from Haiti, Kim was determined to see a doctor for her routine pelvic exam. She'd put off the appointment

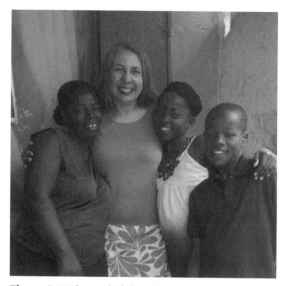

Figure 8.1 Kim and Elvia with Elvia's children, unaware both had cervical cancer

for seven years, allowing her busy life to get in the way. "Finally, I listened to that voice inside me and made myself get my Pap smear." A few days after the test detected abnormal cervical cells, a biopsy revealed Stage 1B cancer. Just as quickly, Kim was referred to an oncologist. In just a "few dizzying days," she started chemoradiation and external beam radiation therapy, followed by brachytherapy.

When Birthplace Becomes a Death Sentence

During her initial treatment, Kim continued working. But three months later, she developed a serious infection in her damaged uterus and needed a hysterectomy. The emotional and surgical ordeal finally took its toll. "I was exhausted," Kim said to me during our September 2020 chat, "so exhausted that I was off work for several months to recover." Like Emily, the Iowan field researcher whose debilitating radiation enteritis precluded her from working, Kim also developed severe radiation enteritis.

"It was awful, so, so awful," she said. "I always had to carry extra clothes in the car because I never knew when I would soil myself." This challenging treatment side effect would continue for three years.

While Kim was undergoing cancer treatment in the United States, in Haiti, Elvia started to experience visible symptoms of cervical cancer, including leg swelling and back pain. Elvia had never had a Pap smear, because in Haiti, Pap smears could cost as much as a month's wages. Screening for cervical cancer is typically infrequent or nonexistent for women there, as it is in many lower-income countries.

Although her treatment was grueling, Kim was grateful for it. She was mortified by the lack of treatment available for Elvia. "They told her that she had a tumor and there was nothing they could do for her," Kim recalled. "At that time, Haiti had no radiation machines in the country, nor did Elvia have any options to access treatment elsewhere."

Indeed, in all of Haiti, no radiation machines are available to provide radiation treatment for cervical cancer; the next closest country for treatment happens to be the United States. During her time in Haiti, Kim learned of profound health care inequities for women. "In Haiti, the rich leave the country to get treatment, the poor have come to expect they will not receive treatment, and the middle-income – well, they may try to raise money to get themselves treated, but their options are very inconsistent." Without that treatment, of course, most Haitian women struck with cervical cancer will die – painfully and quickly.

Kim's experience with this form of inequity became deeply personal. Because Elvia couldn't afford to leave the country for expensive radiation treatment, she died a few months after her diagnosis. "I never saw Elvia again after the visit when that photo was taken," Kim said, her voice laden with sadness. Alongside her grief, Kim was outraged over the injustices her Haitian friend suffered.

"I keep the photo of me and Elvia next to my bed," she told me as she gazed away from the screen, lost in thought. "No matter how painful the brachytherapy was, or how terrible I felt, or how bad the diarrhea was, my kids are going to grow up with my parenting them," she said. "I cannot complain. I am alive. I am alive because I did not live in Haiti. I am alive because I live in a country where I could get treated for cervical cancer. My children still have a mother who is living."

"I am alive. I am alive because I did not live in Haiti. I am alive because I live in a country where I could get treated for cervical cancer. My children still have a mother who is living."

When Kim finally looked at me again, tears rolled down her face. "For no other reasons than where we were born and where we live, Elvia died – and I lived," she said. She shook her head. "I think of that every night when I look at our photo together."

Elvia's kids were ten and eleven when she died.

A Disease of Disparities

Kim's and Elvia's differing journeys point to an ugly paradox. The means to prevent cervical cancer are scientifically sound, and in higher-income countries, usually readily available. As women like Kim know all too well, cervical cancer should be beatable. But in the current global economic and political climate – one that tolerates vast disparities in lifesaving health care – this cancer not only persists but also continues to kill more persons with cervixes every year. As you've already learned, one woman is dying every two minutes of cervical cancer, and that frequency is rising both in the United States and overseas. Given the World Health Organization's recent laser-like focus on the disease and technological leaps in prevention, diagnosis, and treatment, it's worth asking why so many are still dying.

The answer, in a word, is disparities. In the big picture, cervical cancer is largely a disease of disparities. Disparities in health care for women across the globe. Disparities that get in their way of accessing that care, be they financial or geographic barriers, or built-in racial biases in the medical system. Disparities in the provision of knowledge about what kind of care is needed and how to get it. Disparities in who receives a vaccine preventing cervical cancer. Disparities in who can get screened and treated for cervical pre-cancer. Disparities in whose cervical cancer is cured through treatment. Until these disparities can be identified and addressed, women will continue to die of cervical cancer – and they will do so without believing their circumstances can be any different.

Illness Begins with Income Inequity

Cervical cancer is essentially a disease of poor women, with 90 percent of cervical cancer deaths occurring in lower-income countries. A 2020 paper authored by two American researchers offers some insight into the dearth of cervical cancer–fighting services available to the world's most impoverished.[1] These researchers found that while lower-income countries account for 49 percent of the world's population, each government's national health expenditures represent a tiny fraction of overall spending.* Combine these countries' relatively minuscule public health budgets with their higher relative concentrations of disease, and it's easy to see how few funds might be available for sustained cervical cancer screening programs, regardless of burgeoning need.

Indeed, cervical cancer rates show that obstacles to preventing or treating cervical cancer are highest in parts of the world where women struggle to feed themselves and raise their families, places where poverty is the rule rather than the exception. Strategies for preventing deaths via cervical cancer must consider the global inequities that hasten its spread and adapt those

---

* In fact, lower-income countries account for less than 4 percent of total world health spending. By contrast, higher-income countries account for nearly 17 percent of the global population and 81 percent of global health spending. Institute for Health Metrics and Evaluation (IHME), *Financing Global Health 2018: Countries and Programs in Transition.* Seattle, WA: IHME, 2019.

strategies accordingly: addressing everything that gets in the way of women getting the health care they need.

Elvia offers one such example of a woman who died in the absence of essential care. Like so many cervical cancer sufferers, Elvia lived in a country with such limited reproductive health services, she'd lost the fight before she began. Elvia essentially faced three strikes against her future: no HPV vaccine, no screening, and no treatment. It's no wonder cervical cancer continues its quiet rampage across the globe – with no easy way to stop it – despite the overwhelming ability of modern medicine to change that trajectory (Figure 8.2).

Let's Not Forget Racial Inequity

When racial bias intersects with widespread poverty, the results are usually disastrous: greater disease spread, more death. Even a quick glance at a world map of average country income levels shows us that the lowest household incomes are concentrated in typically non-White enclaves in Africa, a continent that also accounts for some of the world's highest rates of cervical cancer (Figure 8.3). Of course, systemic racial bias – the kind that might interfere with equal access to medical privileges – can be nuanced and particular to each race. These biases vary even within those racial groupings, be they Black, Hispanic, Indigenous, or other non-White racial groups. It would be naive to treat a whole race as a monolith and assume all biases are essentially the same. But the research tells us that the economic and political advantages one dominant racial group happens to have over another only amplify the incidence of cervical cancer among the nondominant group. This problem is readily apparent in the world's lower-income countries. It also rears its ugly head in higher-income countries, where women are often marginalized in the health care system for being both poor and non-White.

This correlation between poverty, race, and lack of access to medical care – and the consequent rise in diseases like cervical cancer – is abundantly clear in the United States. According to

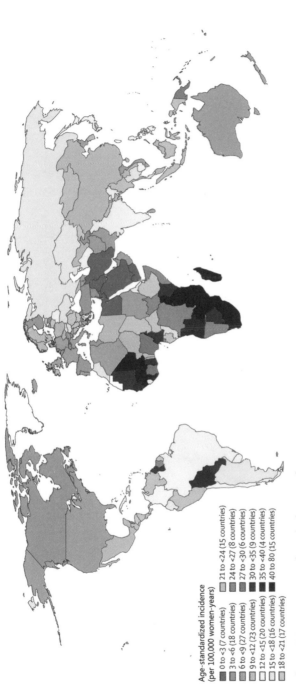

Figure 8.2 New cases of cervical cancer by country

Source: Arbyn, M., E. Weiderpass, L. Bruni, et al. "Estimates of Incidence and Mortality of Cervical Cancer in 2018: A Worldwide Analysis." *Lancet Glob Health* **8**, no. 2 (Feb 2020): e191 -e203. OECD = Organization for Economic Cooperation and Development.

Age-standardized incidence
(per 100,000 women-years)

- 0 to <3 (7 countries)
- 3 to <6 (18 countries)
- 6 to <9 (27 countries)
- 9 to <12 (23 countries)
- 12 to <15 (20 countries)
- 15 to <18 (16 countries)
- 18 to <21 (17 countries)
- 21 to <24 (15 countries)
- 24 to <27 (8 countries)
- 27 to <30 (6 countries)
- 30 to <35 (9 countries)
- 35 to <40 (4 countries)
- 40 to 80 (15 countries)

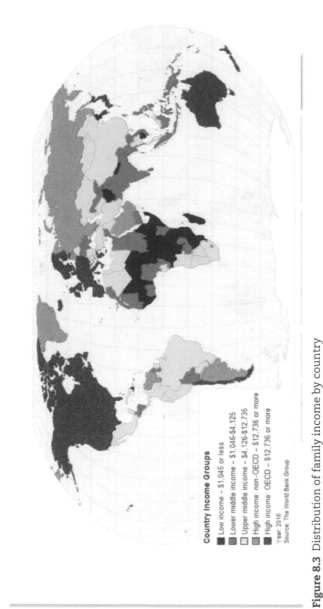

Figure 8.3 Distribution of family income by country

Source: "The World by Income and Region." The World Bank, accessed Jan 29, 2023. https://datatopics.worldbank.org/world-development-indicators/the-world-by-income-and-region.html

2021 data from the Centers for Disease Control and Prevention (CDC), more Black and Hispanic women in the United States get cervical cancer than do White, non-Hispanic women. In every region of the United States, Hispanic women exhibit the highest rates of cervical cancer of *any* racial or ethnic group – 25 percent higher than that of White women.[2] A 2011 U.S.-based study of American Indian and Alaska Native populations found a 60 percent greater rate of cervical cancer among these groups than among non-Indigenous groups.[3] A study published in the 2022 *International Journal of Gynecological Cancer* confirmed the racial divide in cervical cancer incidence between Whites and non-Whites.[4] Again and again, the research reveals a pattern that's racially skewed: cervical cancer disproportionately affects women of color.

Researchers attribute these dangerous disparities to a range of factors, including the absence of sufficient medical providers in lower-income and non-White communities, difficulty obtaining care after abnormal screening results, geographic obstacles to accessing care, distrust of the country's health care system, the lack of targeted messaging for unique cultures and communities, or all of the above. These findings represent a significant hurdle to cervical cancer prevention. Studies indicate that when it comes to eliminating the earliest signs of cervical cancer, non-White, low-income women are missing out on a critical stage of the screening process: after receiving abnormal test results, they're typically not receiving follow-up treatment. In other words, while the system may be doing a passable job in reaching out to disadvantaged women by promoting regular screening appointments or offering subsidized screening clinics and other incentives, it has failed to consider that all-important second step: follow-up to abnormal screening results and treating of pre-cancer to prevent cancer. The implications are monumental. When these women aren't told about the importance of follow-up or given an affordable means of receiving it, they're infinitely more vulnerable to getting advanced cervical cancer.[5] Given the typical barriers these marginalized groups face to getting advanced cancer treatment, they are far more likely to suffer and die as a result.

In the United States, race plays a role not just in how often women are diagnosed with cervical cancer, but also in their likelihood of survival.[6] Consider the fact that five years after a cervical cancer diagnosis, only 58 percent of Black women are still alive, compared with 71 percent of White women, according to the American Society of Clinical Oncology.[7] What's more, U.S. Indian Health Service data recorded between 2009 and 2014 showed that American Indian women and Indigenous women in Alaska had the highest cervical cancer death rates in the country. The stark divide between White and non-White death rates reflects diagnostic differences: cervical cancer is usually diagnosed among non-White women at a more advanced stage, offering a much lower chance of survival.[8] Even though the United States is home to a sophisticated, technologically advanced health care system, underlying inequities and social divisions still get in the way of access to cervical cancer prevention and treatment.

The relationship between inequity and cervical cancer death rates is borne out by a U.S.-based study on survival outcomes for more than 1,500 women with cervical cancer. This twenty-year-old study examined a U.S. military health care system offering its veterans equal access to health care; researchers could control factors like income and access. Conducted when White women with cervical cancer in the U.S. population were 10 to 15 percent more likely to survive cervical cancer than their Black counterparts, the study found that within the equitable veterans' health care system, the margin of survivability disappeared. The authors concluded that when women received cancer care within an equal-access health care system, "Black women's survival can approach that of their non-minority counterparts."[9]

It is outrageous and disheartening to know that a study like this completed two decades ago failed to prompt a public outcry – let alone efforts to equalize cervical cancer rates and outcomes among Black and White women. In more affluent areas of the world, the introduction of the HPV vaccine has begun shrinking the racial divide in cervical cancer rates. HPV vaccination rates are higher among non-White girls and women in the United States, and Black women's pre-cancer rates have begun drawing closer to those of White women, suggesting racial disparities might be diminished by increasingly equitable access to the vaccine. But this positive development has yet to overcome all disparities in race- or income-related cervical cancer rates.

Cervical cancer diagnosis and treatment disparities occur among low-income racial minorities in higher-income countries outside the United States as well. The Australian Institute of Health and Welfare compared cervical cancer diagnoses and survival rates among Australian ethnic groups and found that Indigenous women – typically living on lower incomes in the country's underresourced center – were diagnosed with the disease two and a half times more frequently than non-Indigenous women, and, once diagnosed, Indigenous women were five times more likely to die of their cervical cancer.[10,*] Aboriginal women in Australia may have to travel several hundred miles to reach a clinic providing cervical cancer screening. They are thus less likely to circumvent cancer. This study acknowledged similarly higher rates of cervical cancer and death among Indigenous women in New Zealand and Canada, suggesting that high rates of cervical cancer and mortality may, as the study noted, "be a symptom of social and economic inequity."[*] Roma women, the Indigenous women of Spain and Romania, also show consistently lower cervical cancer screening rates than non-Indigenous women in their respective countries.[11]

Racial and income disparities in cervical cancer survival for Indigenous women remain consistent in countries across the world, a reminder that inequity is, indeed, a global problem.

---

[*] The rate of cervical cancer among women in Australia is 17 per 100,000 in Indigenous women versus 7 per 100,000 in non-Indigenous women. G. D. Shannon, O. H. Franco, J. Powles, Y. Leng, and N. Pashayan, "Cervical Cancer in Indigenous Women: The Case of Australia," *Maturitas* **70**, no. 3 (Nov 2011): 234–45. https://doi.org/10.1016/j.maturitas.2011.07.019 www.ncbi.nlm.nih.gov/pubmed/21889857

These disparities diminish women's survival rates regardless of whether they live in higher-income countries with access to specialized treatment.

While racial inequity is often linked to socioeconomic inequity, it's not always possible to root out inherent biases that get in the way of women's access to health care services. Geographic or cultural barriers, along with a lack of comprehensive medical insurance coverage – affecting persons of any skin color who have cervixes – can independently interfere with cervical cancer care. But our current data indicate that non-White women are more often diagnosed with cervical cancer and more likely to die of it, as are women marginalized for reasons not related to race. It's not too much of a stretch to say that when health care systems are created – intentionally or otherwise – to serve a dominant and privileged population, they hinder nondominant groups from receiving the services they need to prevent or treat a dangerous disease, even when these services are available. We will critically examine these barriers in coming chapters. But there can be no question that acknowledging the long-standing inequities around race and economic status must be part of the overall strategy to eliminate cervical cancer.

Geographic Inequity: A Bigger Factor Than Expected

Geographic barriers also get in the way of access to reproductive health care to a degree many find surprising. Within a single country, even, cervical cancer rates can vary wildly within regions or territories.

Between 2010 and 2014, the CDC compared diagnostic efficacy within different geographic locations and races and found that rural women had higher rates of every stage of cervical cancer than did their urban or White counterparts.[12] This disparity in cancer rates according to geography – where a woman lives – is influenced by a number of factors: her income level (typically lower in rural regions), the topography of the region (such as mountainous regions with poor roads), and access issues (including a lack of health care providers or lack of clinics in rural areas). In this way, geographic inequity can impede early cancer care and diagnoses for women in the same way race does.

These factors translate to a system of unequal access to the means of preventing cervical cancer – especially for non-White women in remote or rural areas – and only reinforce the difficulty of eliminating the disease.

The Hidden Toll of Financial Inequity

While it's tempting to assume the vast majority of inequity in health care happens in lower-income countries, in wealthier parts of the world such as the United States, women's ability to cover their own health care costs varies widely based on income and access to comprehensive medical insurance. In the absence of universal health care systems found in countries like the United Kingdom, Australia, and Canada – systems that cover the majority of citizens' medical expenses – heated debates about subsidizing certain health care services have persisted for years in individual U.S. states. The country's sharp, internal divisions are readily apparent. Its system of private insurance mixed with inconsistent access to care creates a fearsome inequity for persons with cervixes – one largely based on the state in which they happen to live.

Over the years, politically motivated or ill-informed state legislatures have also declined to expand their Medicaid programs, which come with federal funding and greater access to cervical cancer care, among many other things. Reduction in Medicaid support has resulted in closures of women's health clinics across the country, dramatically restricting access to female reproductive services. A 2019 study of state clinic closures between 2010 and 2013 found a consequent, yet unsurprising, decline in cervical cancer screenings, with the highest decrease among socially marginalized groups: Hispanic women's screening rates dropped almost 6 percent; women aged twenty-one to thirty-four showed a drop of more than 5 percent; unmarried women's screening rates dropped more than 4 percent; and uninsured patients' screening rates plummeted almost 7 percent. As a result, the number of women diagnosed with early-stage cervical cancer decreased by 13 percent – not because cervical cancer rates went down, but because more women were diagnosed at a later stage and thus 36 percent more likely to die of cervical cancer.[13]

The cost of care and the absence of medical insurance appear to play a key role in women's willingness to take part in cervical cancer prevention. In 2018, a research group at MD Anderson Cancer Hospital examined this issue in the Rio Grande Valley and Laredo regions located along the Texas–Mexico border. Among a population of 1.5 million, researchers found that about 70,000 females aged twenty-one to sixty-five – the prime age for cervical cancer screening – lacked insurance coverage. As a result, their participation in screening was abysmal: only 13 percent received the necessary Pap tests or follow-up care.[14]

The Texas study noted systemic barriers to screening, including publicly funded clinics with insufficient health care providers and a clear deficit in the clinical capacity to serve them. Some women lacked an understanding of the critical importance of cervical screening. These women were typically struggling to work, feed their children, care for elderly family members, and run a household rather than focus on their own health needs. They cited a range of reasons for not getting screened, including being unable to miss work or find transportation to a local clinic or being afraid of deportation through registering as a patient. Overall, 87 percent of those women – almost 60,000 – were forgoing screening for cervical cancer, a rate comparable to lower-income countries like Zimbabwe or Mongolia.

The defunding of Planned Parenthood clinics in some U.S. states – a trend expected to escalate in the wake of the 2022 constitutional reversal on abortion rights – has obstructed the ability of low-income or uninsured women to access basic reproductive health care. These cuts directly interfere with cervical cancer care. Planned Parenthood alone sees roughly 3 million U.S. women annually and performs 500,000 Pap tests every year. And yet, state politicians have been whittling away at these services for more than a decade. In 2011, Wisconsin state governor Scott Walker signed a bill eliminating all state funding for Planned Parenthood, which contributed to the closure of five rural clinics. In Texas, Planned Parenthood clinics were a primary target for the 2011 pro-life legislature's funding cuts, including clinics that provided only contraceptive and sexually transmitted infection services, and no abortion at all. Women's health was again on the chopping block in 2015, when the Texas legislature blocked Planned Parenthood clinics from participating in a state-run program providing breast cancer and cervical cancer screenings for women on a low income. In the Gulf Coast region of the state, Planned Parenthood cuts affected screenings for more than 13,000 women, many of them in areas with limited health care alternatives.[15] In communities where Planned Parenthood is the only provider of affordable Pap smears, this sort of legislative action is simply government-supported inequity.

The results of a new University of California in Los Angeles study published in June 2022 shed a disturbing light on the possible fallout of ongoing, state-by-state budget cuts to reproductive health care. Their findings? Advanced cervical cancer cases are actually increasing in the United States.[5] The consequences are being felt in the southern states in particular, where clinic closures or refusals for Medicaid expansion appear most apt to take place. The California-based research team evaluated the U.S. National Cancer Institute's database of all cervical cancer cases diagnosed between 2001 and 2018, and determined that while Black and Hispanic women continued to report the highest number of advanced cervical cancer diagnoses, Southern White women showed the highest increase in Stage 4 cervical cancer rates. They attributed these increases to high numbers of women who couldn't afford to get regularly screened or weren't told why it was important, as well as numerous White teenage girls eschewing the HPV vaccine.

It's alarming enough to see advanced cervical cancer rates soaring in a country as wealthy as the United States, but when our health policies either overlook, actively discourage, or diminish prevention options for young, poor, or non-White women, it does not bode well for efforts to do away with this disease.

Information Inequity: The Message Missing the Mark

In addition to detecting geographic health care hurdles women faced on the Texas–Mexico border, the 2018 MD Anderson Cancer Hospital study zeroed in on women's distrust of the medical system and the government.[14] Many of the region's residents reported not feeling safe to show up for appointments without fear of deportation. These women heard an unspoken message against "foreigners" – perpetuated by communal fears and suspicions – and they opted out of care as a result. Messaging matters.

As politically motivated state legislatures continue to restrict women's reproductive health services through health clinic closures, U.S. women have received another powerful message: their health is simply not valued. When women on low incomes of all skin colors lose out on subsidized cervical cancer screening, they forgo this crucial form of disease prevention. Ill-considered changes in health care policy instantly put vulnerable women at risk of getting and dying of cervical cancer. And the insinuation is always: you matter less than other women. You are not worth care.

Overt messaging about clinic closures or implied threats of deportation are not the only way we communicate about women's health. Women's perceptions are powerfully shaped by the voices of everyone in their sphere, including subtle and unspoken cues about the benefits of services like cervical cancer screening, or widespread and vocal discouragement against HPV vaccination. A multicountry study looking at cervical cancer screening rates among Southeast Asian women who immigrated to Canada and the United Kingdom (as well as the United States) found that inherent belief systems made these women skeptical about preventative health measures and culturally averse to pelvic examinations.[16] When public health messaging fails to consider others' beliefs or education about health care, it becomes another barrier to prevention. Public health messaging must include *all* women and address the concerns of *all* women, or it is just another inequity getting in the way of stopping cervical cancer.

"Equity-Resilient" Health Care

Competing priorities in health care and finite public health care space will always pose challenges for any country; established cervical cancer care is no different. As we've all seen, unanticipated global health emergencies – such as a pandemic – can divert attention away from other important causes. During the peak of COVID-19, for instance, fewer women worldwide sought or received screening for cervical cancer because of social distancing constraints and soaring demands on health care systems. The COVID-19 pandemic exacerbated disparities for women relying on subsidized clinics or living in areas of the world struggling to provide widespread cervical cancer screening.[17] In many countries, the pandemic revealed the fragile state of funding decisions about reproductive health care services.[18-20]

Rather than bemoaning the distraction away from fighting cervical cancer, we can see these post-pandemic revelations as a welcome opportunity to make our health care systems more "equity-resilient." In other words, it will take heated and persistent advocacy at both the grassroots and government levels to keep the cervical cancer elimination effort at the forefront, especially when challenges like the COVID-19 pandemic may be repeated in future. This pandemic exposed our vulnerability as a global community, magnifying the plight of society's most disenfranchised while showing how disease can be immune to privilege.

We've seen how much we depend on each other to conquer viruses or cancers on a global level. By understanding our interconnectedness, we can begin to strip away ongoing inequities in health care, knowing that doing so is for the benefit of all. We can take a hard look at the inequities that killed Elvia (and continue to torment Kim), and make righting the balance our common cause.

9 LOSING THE LIFE LOTTERY BECAUSE OF WHERE YOU ARE BORN

Picture this: You work for the ministry of health in a country the World Bank classifies as "lower-income." Against a country-wide backdrop of poverty, you feel privileged to have a job you love, and you're passionate about making a difference for fellow citizens – whose average family earns less than $1,500 USD a year and for whom the government can allocate annual health spending of just $75 USD per person.

Cervical cancer is the leading cause of cancer deaths among women in your country, and you've felt that loss acutely. Among your community's loss of countless other mothers, grandmothers, aunties, and sisters, your own Auntie Zena died just last year of cervical cancer at forty-one. You now care for her three daughters in addition to your four sons, and you feel, ever so keenly, the burden of these losses. What you wouldn't give to ensure your three new daughters are never diagnosed with cervical cancer.

No wonder your ears prick up when you hear your country might be eligible for the HPV vaccine through funding from the international aid organization known as Gavi. Because of your work, you're familiar with this miraculous vaccine and the Geneva-based global health partnership that helps provide it to lower-income countries. If Gavi is involved, your country might have a chance to end cervical cancer the way it ended polio so many decades ago.

You roll up your sleeves and get to work. You plan meticulously. In keeping with World Health Organization recommendations, you propose vaccination of all nine- to fourteen-year-old girls in the first year of vaccine introduction and craft a plan for universal, ongoing vaccination of all nine-year-old girls after that. You know your country faces logistical challenges in delivering the vaccine – the actual "shots in arms" – having had little experience in vaccine distribution to older children and preteens. To counter this problem, you work with community and education leaders to devise a school-delivery model that allows for maximum reach.

You calculate how many refrigerators and freezers you'll need for vaccine storage, and how to safely transport the vaccine, which must be kept cold, across your blistering hot country. You outline complex logistics for vaccination in villages, many of which lack electrical power. You consider how to engage community leaders, school officials, women's groups, social media influencers, and religious leaders to endorse and actively promote the vaccine to girls and their parents, taking into consideration the highly charged gender issues around vaccinating only girls in your traditional, male-dominated society, and how to address misinformation campaigns that might derail the entire project. Your goal is nothing less than a country-wide vaccination rollout achieving "herd immunity" within a few years. You want 90 percent of the population vaccinated to stop HPV transmission – thwarting cervical cancer in your country.

After hundreds of hours of work, you submit your application to Gavi for consideration and are rewarded a few months later with the joyous news that your application has been approved! You have secured doses for all nine- to fourteen-year-old girls in your country for the first year, as well as all nine-year-old girls in future years. You know the estimate that one case of cervical cancer can be prevented by vaccination of just seventy girls.[1] With these data in mind, plus the promised doses and completion of your plan, you celebrate: Auntie Zena's daughters will surely escape their mother's fate and live free of the threat of death from cervical cancer.

> You know the estimate that one case of cervical cancer can be prevented by vaccination of just seventy girls.

And then, another letter from Gavi arrives with news that is – in this part of the world – neither surprising nor uncommon. "Dear Farai, we are sorry to inform you," Gavi writes, "of a current supply constraint of the HPV vaccine." Gavi cannot secure the doses you asked for. You will have to delay HPV vaccine introduction for at least a year, maybe two, and even then, you will only have enough to vaccinate your country's nine-year-olds.

Your heart breaks. Your daughters and other girls whose lives you'd hoped to change have now likely missed their chance for this vaccine. Perhaps your country's nine-year-olds will be vaccinated in a few years, but thousands of girls have just lost a cruel "life lottery." In the meantime, the global HPV vaccine supply will continue finding its way to higher-income countries that can afford the market price. But you and other countries relying on Gavi for the leverage, negotiation, and partnerships to get any vaccines at all will just have to wait.

Vaccination Relies on the Whims of the Marketplace

I've seen this dispiriting – and, in a global context, alarming – scenario play out again and again among countries forced to compete for scarce medical resources. At $31,000 USD per person for the first year after diagnosis in a higher-income country like Canada, the high cost of cervical cancer treatment means it simply isn't available to women in lower-income countries. In places like these, vaccination and screening are not just cost-effective options for avoiding cervical cancer – they are the *only* options. And yet, those costs can be prohibitive. The HPV vaccine is subject to the laws of supply and demand like any other global product. When supply of the vaccine is tight, it keeps a stranglehold on price – and thereby, affordability. The countries most able to benefit from the vaccine become those least able to pay for it.

Keep in mind that the United States has been offering the HPV vaccine for more than fifteen years. A couple of years after U.S. approval of the vaccine in 2006, seventy countries around the world had gone on to approve it. And by 2008, countries with robust public health budgets were ratcheting up the war on cervical cancer. But for countries in the lower-income world – those with the highest burden of cervical cancer, meager public health budgets, and ailing national health care systems – the long wait for a ticket to a cruel life lottery began.

In more affluent global regions, countries have their own regulatory agency, such as the Food and Drug Administration (FDA) for the United States, or they share a regulatory agency (Europe has its European Medicines Agency, for example), that governs access to the vaccine. For higher-income countries, these agencies maintain a consistent, regular flow of HPV vaccine approvals. Lower-income countries, however, typically lack the resources and expertise to have their own regulatory agencies. Instead, these countries rely on the World Health Organization (WHO) to review safety data and approve and recommend vaccines. While the WHO's rigorous process ensures countries receive safe, high-quality HPV vaccines, it implies longer wait times. Given the strict age ranges associated with cancer prevention, any delays can translate to hundreds of thousands of girls missing out on sparing themselves cervical cancer.

Countries Deemed "Too Rich" for Vaccine Funding

In 2009, the WHO offered its worldwide endorsement of the HPV vaccine and recommended it for all girls nine through fourteen. International aid organizations like UNICEF and Gavi needed this WHO "prequalification" before they could purchase the vaccine on behalf of lower-income countries. The WHO's prequalification process is just one example of the steps required to make the vaccine available to countries that can't afford it.

By 2012, Gavi had negotiated $4.55 USD per dose on behalf of its donor countries, making fifty-three countries with the lowest annual gross domestic product eligible for the vaccine. With funding now possible, these countries began the laborious process you imagined at the beginning of this chapter: crafting plans for vaccine delivery they would submit to Gavi for HPV vaccine approval and funding. A full seven years later, by 2019, just eighteen of those fifty-three Gavi-eligible countries had launched their national HPV vaccination programs.

What a striking dichotomy! Within a year of vaccine introduction, girls in the United States and Australia had gotten their "shots in arms," but countries like Cameroon and Cambodia – forced to wait for lower prices and funding – took another thirteen years to do the same. Thirteen years in which their young girls remained entirely at the mercy of a killer virus. Lives lost for an initial investment of less than five U.S. dollars per person.[*]

Consider the fact that girls in Gavi-eligible countries are the "lucky ones," because here's the killer conundrum: while many lower-income countries receive subsidies, an entire cohort of countries in the middle get left out altogether – too "rich" for Gavi funding but lacking the public health monies to support a national HPV vaccine program. I call these the "caught-in-the-middle" countries.

Countries that don't meet the Gavi threshold can negotiate the price – if they're in a position to negotiate. In South America, the Pan American Health Organization has facilitated the bulk purchase of the vaccine for its member countries for

---

[*] When lower-income countries are considering affordability of the HPV vaccine, they'll need to factor into the market price the costs associated with vaccine delivery. Delivery to appropriate age groups can be challenging, because the HPV vaccine cannot rely on the delivery systems used to provide early childhood vaccines. K. Vaughan, A. Ozaltin, M. Mallow, *et al.*, "The Costs of Delivering Vaccines in Low- and Middle-Income Countries: Findings from a Systematic Review," *Vaccine X* **2** (Aug 9 2019): 100034. www .ncbi.nlm.nih.gov/pubmed/31428741

$10 USD.[2] That's almost twice what Gavi pays for the vaccine, but it's far, far less than the $160 USD countries like the United States pay for it. Even for countries deemed too well off for Gavi funding, the average negotiated non-group rate of $11.59 USD per vaccine presents a tremendous barrier. Remember that even these "middling" countries typically have small health care budgets and competing health needs. A 2019 WHO HPV vaccine global market study revealed that the HPV vaccine can account for up to 56 percent of a country's total vaccine expenditure.[3] Namibia is one of those countries caught in the middle.

Namibia: The Best-Laid Plans Won't Pay for Prevention

In the fall of 2017, after a forty-hour journey over three continents, my plane hit the tarmac in Namibia's capital city, Windhoek, located in the country's vast central region. This was my first time working as a physician policy advisor in this southwestern African country, and despite numbing jet lag and swollen ankles, I was sincerely thankful to have been asked to come. I was there to help the Namibian health ministry improve the delivery of cervical cancer screening. My service on the WHO's steering committee for cervical cancer screening guidelines was of value to this nation of almost 3 million, where the average life span is sixty-eight years and cervical cancer is second only to breast cancer as the most common cancer-killer of women.[4]

The eighteen miles from the airport to my hotel featured sparse, windswept vegetation clinging to dry sand that gave way to blue-tinted mountains in the distance, all against a cloudless, deep azure sky. I was reminded of the landscape of Wyoming where I grew up. My professional task here in Namibia was not new to me, either: assisting the ministry of health as they improved their plans for cervical cancer screening. Women in Namibia were suffering and dying, and even without a comprehensive cancer tracking system, the Namibian health ministry was aware of this alarming statistic: in some regions, more than 25 percent of reproductive-aged women were HIV-positive, and, as noted in Chapter 7, this fact had profoundly accelerated the country's rate of cervical cancer. I was there to offer guidance in building a robust screening program identifying women with HPV before they developed cancer, and I knew my Namibian colleagues were desperate for the same outcome.

As I was soon to hear, again and again, they were also desperate for the vaccine. During my stay, I was peppered with questions – "What about this HPV vaccine everyone is talking about? Why can't we gain better access to that?" – and would learn that two years prior to my arrival, the local health ministry had developed a vaccine delivery plan for the same reasons they had invited me to support their screening program: too many women were dying. I was impressed by their ardent enthusiasm and meticulous rollout plan. They had outlined strategies to find, track, and deliver vaccines, even in rural and remote areas of the country. They had set reasonable goals and outlined creative public messaging plans, even preparing ahead of time for inevitable rumors and misinformation. My colleagues weren't asking me how to implement a vaccine rollout. They were asking me how to get the vaccine.

These visionaries – committed, diligent people – just wanted an easily administered injection that higher-income countries had been using for eleven years. Their simple desire turned out to be not so simple. I was discouraged to confront the reality that cost was the final barrier for cancer prevention in Namibia. Thankfully, a recent intervention from the United Nations has offered the country a ray of hope. In November 2022, the Namibian government approved procurement of the quadrivalent HPV vaccine through the support of the UN International Children's Fund. It plans to offer the vaccine to 20 percent of its nine- to fourteen-year-old girls in the first year, increasing to 70 percent over three years.[5] All of which is welcome news, but unfortunately doesn't offer guarantees the country will be able to finance an expensive, long-range HPV vaccine plan to protect girls in the future from cervical cancer–causing HPV. Even in countries the World Bank has deemed "high income" – with a gross national income per capita[6] of $13,205 USD or more in 2022 – the HPV vaccine price tag can be daunting. When it was initially offered in the United States, the vaccine cost roughly $120 USD per dose (before it jumped another $40 USD when the newer, HPV-9 vaccine came to market). These figures still don't account for the ancillary costs of office visits and injection administration, all making for a pricy investment of public health dollars.

As a point of comparison, the annual flu vaccine costs $25 USD[7] and a child's tetanus/diphtheria/pertussis vaccine just $20 USD.[8] In countries with universal, government-funded health care, like England, Sweden, and Canada, for example, persons with cervixes have their vaccines paid for. But in the United States, we have our own "caught-in-the-middle" populations. Girls eighteen and younger from lower-income families on subsidized health care plans such as Medicaid are vaccinated for free via the federally sponsored Vaccines for Children program. Families with private insurance may also have free or reduced-cost vaccines. But for those "caught in the middle," with no insurance or limited coverage, the HPV vaccine remains as out of reach as it does for the girls of Namibia. Another cruel ticket in a lousy lottery.

Vaccine Supplies No Match for Crushing Demand

None of us is unfamiliar with this inhumane system, where those who can afford to live get to live, and those who can't, don't. You may be one of those "caught-in-the-middle" people like so many of my patients who struggle to receive adequate care in the world's wealthiest country, because they don't have enough insurance – or any at all. And we have all just lived through the worst of a pandemic where a lifesaving vaccine available to everyone in higher-income countries has been desperately slow to reach the vast majority of lower-income countries.

It behooves us as a society to address this bizarre arrangement – assigning value to a human life based on residency – for reasons relating to cervical cancer and beyond. But here's the dark secret behind letting market forces decide whether or not a girl gets the HPV vaccine and, by extension, protection from cervical cancer. Until recently, a single company produced the vast majority of the HPV vaccine's global supply. Yes, you read that right: Merck & Co, Inc., an American company based in New Jersey, has been the predominant supplier of the vaccine. Added to Merck's near-monopoly on supply is the fact that this company recently struggled to meet global HPV vaccine demand. The result – as if barriers like cost and regulatory processes weren't enough – has been a global supply shortage since 2018. That's four years when the crass laws of supply and demand were allowed to straitjacket thousands of cervical cancer prevention opportunities.

After HPV vaccine deliveries were delayed to an estimated twenty-nine lower-income countries, the WHO's Strategic Advisory Group of Experts (SAGE) called for a policy change to address a supply crisis.* SAGE proposed two strategies. First, in 2019, it asked all countries to temporarily discontinue HPV vaccination for girls over fifteen and for boys.[9] Second, SAGE asked countries to target the vaccine only toward a single age group of girls – only nine- or ten-year-old girls, for instance – contrary to its 2017 recommendation that all nine- to fourteen-year-old girls receive the vaccine in the first year of introduction. By April 2022, and in response to trials showing HPV vaccine effectiveness after just a single dose, SAGE added a further strategy, recommending countries alter their approach by offering single HPV vaccine doses to all nine- to fourteen-year-olds.[10]

---

* SAGE = a group of independent global experts charged with advising WHO on global policy and strategies.

These strategies maximized vaccine supply while easing pressure on demand: undervaccinated countries required fewer HPV vaccine doses but could still protect larger age ranges of girls. Developments such as these offered encouraging news for countries relying solely on vaccination to prevent cervical cancer. As of June 2022, Dr. Kate O'Brien, WHO Director of the Department of Immunization, Vaccines and Biologicals, reported a steady improvement in global supply constraints on the HPV vaccine.

But HPV vaccine use has lost ground following a two-year-plus focus on the global COVID-19 pandemic. What's more, when SAGE introduced its vaccine-sparing strategy in 2019, some lower-income countries – unable to procure any HPV vaccines in the midst of a global shortage – had to halt introduction of HPV vaccination altogether.[11] "Currently, only thirteen percent of the world's nine- to fourteen-year-olds are receiving the HPV vaccine," Dr. O'Brien said. "And these are often not in the countries that make up the heavy cervical cancer burden." Improvement of the HPV vaccine programs, she said, remains at the top of the WHO's agenda. "Of all the vaccines used, HPV vaccines and measles are the two vaccines that provide the biggest gains in preventing deaths."

For now, though, lower-income countries bear the brunt of high prices and insufficient vaccine supply. Higher-income countries, meanwhile, have not only ensured their recommended age groups were inoculated, but have also expanded HPV vaccination to a wider age range of females and to boys. According to UNICEF's most recent "Human Papillomavirus: Supply and Demand Update," higher-income countries account for 69 percent of global vaccine supply, compared with a 13 percent share accorded lower-income countries. Amid this strain on resources, a 2022 WHO Global Market Study shows that boys account for one-tenth of vaccine use,[3] despite tracing the number of HPV cancers in males globally to just under 60,000 cancer cases. By contrast, the HPV virus has been linked annually to more than 570,000 cancer cases in women.[12-14]

While it would be ideal to eliminate all HPV-related cancers, it makes sense amid a global HPV vaccine shortage to focus first on the gender with the most significant cancer burden. This tactic promises to ultimately benefit boys by reducing HPV-16 prevalence in girls, thereby reducing the risk of its sexual transmission to boys.[15,16]

In the meantime, prospective new sources of increased HPV vaccine production suggest good news on the anti–cervical cancer front. Merck has plans to build two new manufacturing facilities, a Chinese manufacturer has recently developed an approved HPV vaccine, and India is working on its own as well: all factors expected to alleviate supply shortages by 2024.[2,17]

Expanded supply of the vaccine offers reassurance for future generations, but implies sticking the current generation of girls with the "who-gets-to-live lottery": the status quo. As a result of HPV vaccine supply constraints, Gavi estimates that, between 2021 and 2025, 34 million girls will have missed out on being immunized against HPV.[18] At a rate of needing to vaccinate 70 girls to prevent a single case of cervical cancer, supply constraints will have caused nearly 500,000 more cases of cervical cancer. That's enough girls to fill a medium-sized city, enough women to fill the largest soccer stadium in the world four times over. Enough? Too many. Far, far too many.

At a rate of needing to vaccinate 70 girls to prevent a single case of cervical cancer, supply constraints will have caused nearly 500,000 more cases of cervical cancer.

Nigeria: A Country with No HPV Vaccine Supply

While some countries struggle to vaccinate their girls against cervical cancer, supply-chain economics strips many lower-income nations of their defenses altogether. Nigeria, a vibrant west African country with a population of 217 million – more people than Australia, Canada, the United Kingdom, and France combined[19] – effectively has no supply of the HPV vaccine. Added to the absence of this most potent source of cervical cancer prevention is the fact that Nigeria is home to high rates of HIV. Roughly 3.2 million Nigerians have been diagnosed with HIV, with fifteen- to forty-nine-year-old Nigerian women three times more likely than same-aged men to be HIV-positive.[20] In light of HIV's accelerant effect on HPV, the absence of an HPV vaccine lays Nigerian women bare to developing cervical cancer.

During a July 2022 International Federation of Gynaecology and Obstetrics (FIGO) conference on improving HPV vaccine use in lower-income countries, I met the First Lady of Niger State, Dr. Amina Abubakar Bello. A practicing obstetrician, gynecologist, and public health physician, Dr. Bello told me that her country's modest health care budget had typically made HPV vaccination available only to Nigerian girls whose families could afford to buy it themselves. A more recent global shortage and Nigeria's low ranking on manufacturers' priority lists has significantly diminished the country's access to the vaccine. As a result, Dr. Bello said that privately funded access to the vaccine in Nigeria has all but disappeared. "It breaks my heart to know that cervical cancer should not happen. And yet we watch it flourish without [the HPV vaccine] in our country."

Wanted: A Global Vision for Vaccination

In 2019, the CDC's Advisory Committee on Immunization Practices (the ACIP, which, in full disclosure, I serve on as a non-voting liaison representing the American College of Obstetricians and Gynecologists) approved a proposal to add twenty-seven- to forty-five-year-old women and men to its list of HPV vaccine-eligible candidates, even though the cancer-fighting benefits are vastly lower for older recipients. Since the fall of 2020, I regularly receive emails from Merck encouraging me to recommend the HPV vaccine to my female patients up to age forty-five. In the face of a global shortage and inequitable distribution of the HPV vaccine, these emails – and the developments they reflect – disturb me deeply as a practitioner.

I have seen firsthand what cervical cancer vaccination can do for a girl in a lower-income country, where treatment is unavailable, and a diagnosis of cervical cancer is a death sentence – pure and simple. In a highly resourced country like the United States, where cervical cancer screening programs exist, it takes 6,500 vaccinations of women aged forty to prevent one case of cervical cancer.[21] By contrast, when the vaccine is given to girls at nine before they're sexually active – and in a country like Nigeria or Namibia lacking routine screening – only seventy of those girls need vaccination to prevent a single case. As a physician who tries to offer equitable care, I find these statistics hard to ignore.

Former ACIP voting member Dr. Kelly Moore, a public health and vaccine expert from Tennessee, voted against the 2019 plan to expand age eligibility for the HPV vaccine. I spoke with her about her rationale for opposing the vaccine for older women and men. "What I found particularly upsetting following that ACIP meeting," she told me, "was being at the SAGE meeting just a few months later when there were seven presentations over several hours evaluating different scenarios for stretching the tiny supply of HPV vaccine across as many eligible nine- to fourteen-year-old girls in as many [lower-income] countries as possible to save as many lives as possible." For Dr. Moore, the ACIP and SAGE discussions demonstrated global stewards of public health trying to minimize death from two very different perspectives. Both had good intentions, but one was focused on protecting U.S. citizens, and another kept a bird's-eye view on global health equity. The ACIP vote supported offering the HPV vaccine to women and men up to age forty-five in the United States. One wonders how different the outcome might have been had ACIP members first attended the SAGE presentation and been able to ponder the larger implications of reducing cervical cancer worldwide.

As a gynecologist caring for women in the United States, I know many of my colleagues, as well as my patients, are unaware of the global HPV vaccine shortage. They have little idea how desperately the world's poorest countries would like to protect their young girls against the ravages of cervical cancer. Personally, I wrestle with this knowledge every time one of my patients sits in front of me asking if she should consider the vaccine. When a forty-year-old, newly divorced patient, for instance, comes in to talk about HPV vaccination to protect her from new sexual partners, I will caution her about its relative limitations for a woman her age. "The HPV vaccine can help protect you from acquiring a new HPV infection," I will say, "providing the vaccine offers protection for that HPV type, and when it's an HPV type you've not been exposed to before."* I will also tell her that the HPV vaccine provides much lower efficacy for her than it would for a nine-year-old girl. "Keep in mind the likelihood that you've already acquired an HPV infection." Together, my patient and I will discuss the pros and cons and make a decision either way. Yet, throughout these discussions, my global citizen heart is also speaking to me, and I feel torn – especially when I consider the value of offering this precious resource to the thousands of nine-year-old girls in countries offering no cervical screening, and no cervical cancer treatment once it develops.

Until vaccine shortages are examined through a global lens, girls and women in lower-income countries will continue to be shortchanged on preventing cervical cancer. And they will continue to die: the losers in a barbaric lottery system. I celebrate the expected reduction in global supply constraints over the next few years. But as long as vaccination costs remain out of reach, the terrible truth of "where you live means whether you live" will take its toll on persons with cervixes worldwide.

In recent years, I watched with amazement as global governments funded rapid COVID-19 vaccine development and

---

* Receiving the nonavalent HPV vaccine would protect my patient against HPV types 6, 11, 16, 18, 31, 33, 45, 52, and 58 (the HPV strains that the vaccine can protect against) if she had not previously been exposed to these strains. National Cancer Institute, "Recombinant Human Papillomavirus (HPV) Nonavalent Vaccine," updated March 10, 2023. www.cancer.gov/about-cancer/treatment/drugs/recombinant-hpv-nonavalent-vaccine.

production amid an economy-crushing pandemic. Most of us celebrated when COVID-19 vaccines first became available in late 2020, and at that time, vaccinating 80 to 120 people prevented a single case of COVID-19 (an illness from which the vast majority recover).[22] By contrast, it only takes seventy HPV vaccinations given to girls in countries that lack screening to prevent a case of cervical cancer, when cervical cancer is all too often a death sentence. I wonder why the epidemic of cervical cancer – for which a vaccine has been available for nearly two decades – continues unabated.

A lousy lottery, indeed.

10 SEX, LIES, AND LOGISTICS: OBSTACLES TO VACCINATION BEYOND THE MARKETPLACE

For an injection that's just a quick jab in the arm, entry of the HPV vaccine into the postmodern world has been anything but pain-free. Public perceptions – many of them misperceptions – have a lot to do with widespread resistance to its use. Consider the case of Japan. As a country with one of the highest initial uptakes of the vaccine, Japan's HPV vaccination campaign was deemed a huge success. In fact, when the HPV vaccine was approved for use in 2009, the island nation of almost 126 million quickly leapt to the front of the line. An astonishing 70 percent of girls twelve to sixteen got vaccinated.

But in 2013, Japanese media began publishing sensational reports of adverse symptoms to the vaccine, such as fainting, fever, pain, even muscle disorders, and over the next three years, the national HPV vaccination rate dropped like a stone: from 74 percent to less than 1 percent. Despite Japanese-based safety studies that found no evidence of vaccine-related side effects, anxious politicians suspended the campaign, fear and rumors robbing an entire generation of Japanese girls of near-perfect protection against a killer cancer.

From Hero to Zero in Just One Year

It was only in 2022, after much activism on the part of Japanese physicians, researchers, and survivors – including Junko Mihara, a prominent elected official and women's health activist – that the country's government decided to restart the HPV vaccination program.[1] I was one of many rejoicing at the news. At the same time, I decried the fact that this rejuvenated campaign arrived too late for the estimated 10,000 Japanese women expected to develop cervical cancer every year, and the 3,000 who die annually from the disease.[2]

Those of us who watched the panic, paranoia, and propaganda swirl against a fierce global push for COVID-19 vaccination might detect the eerie similarities with Japan and the HPV vaccine. What can seem like a simple, sensible health intervention – a shot that prevents a killer virus – becomes a social, cultural, religious, and political football, tossed around like a game: a deadly game, where lives are at stake.

Hesitancy, Suspicion, and Outright Fear

We already know that the fight to end cervical cancer faces mighty obstacles around cost and supply. But, like the immunization campaign to stop COVID-19, vaccination efforts against the HPV virus must contend with the bigger enemy of public perception. Think of the frenzy created concerning large-scale immunization programs, and then try to track its origins. More often, widespread anti-vax sentiment has little to do with science. It starts with good old-fashioned misinformation, widely circulated, and then amped up by social media. A solution designed to tackle a public health emergency gets repackaged as a diabolical way for government to control its citizens.

With regard to the HPV vaccine, fear-fueled disinformation campaigns have allowed its use to be associated with painful side effects, and even tragic outcomes. These claims directly contradict the findings of hundreds of scientists and the world's top safety monitoring agencies. Researchers have published

more than 1,300 articles on HPV vaccine safety since it was first
licensed, issuing 180 safety reports in the first 6 months of 2021
alone. Global and national safety groups, like the Global
Advisory Committee on Vaccine Safety, which reports to the
WHO, the U.S.-based Centers for Disease Control and
Prevention (CDC), and Sweden's Uppsala Monitoring Centre
have extensively and repeatedly studied and affirmed the safety
of the HPV vaccine. Moreover, more than 280 million doses
have been delivered worldwide, and not one public health
monitoring system has unearthed a related pattern of serious
side effects.

Despite the HPV vaccine's enviable safety record, hesitancy,
suspicion, and outright fear continue to challenge public health
ministries and agencies, hobbling their efforts at timely and
universal uptake of a lifesaving prevention measure. In India,
which in 2020 had 75,000 cervical cancer cases (or 12 percent of
the global burden[3]) and a dense population struggling to provide screening, the HPV vaccine seemed like the means to
vanquish a potent killer. Instead, its debut in India ground to
a halt. In 2009, a demonstration project designed to vaccinate
nearly 25,000 girls against HPV was suspended after the press
falsely attributed six deaths to the vaccine. A local investigation
revealed the various causes of death to be a poisonous snake
bite, drowning in a quarry, a high fever from malaria, and
suicide, but public anxiety halted the project.[4] It was 2016
before the HPV vaccine could be used for privately paying
patients in New Delhi,[5] and India as a whole has yet to offer
widespread vaccination. When ill-timed poisonous reactions,
seizures, and even death are attributed to HPV vaccination,
health care providers and public health officials are hard-
pressed to find the time, energy, and money to respond appro-
priately to the resulting public outcry.

Every country, whether lower- or higher-income, is susceptible to public disinformation campaigns, and the United
States is no exception. Since its introduction, the HPV vaccine
has been subjected to a lot of negative U.S. press, partly
accounting for its slow uptake. Among the most damaging of

these reports featured former presidential candidate and congresswoman Michele Bachmann and television talk show host Katie Couric, both of whom offered public platforms to parents linking the HPV vaccine to tragic outcomes. In 2011, Bachmann shared on television the story of a mother who believed the vaccine caused developmental disabilities in her daughter. In 2013, Couric hosted a mother who claimed the vaccine led to her daughter's death. In both instances, neither of these powerful public figures substantiated the grief-stricken parents' claims or countered them with information about vaccine safety or efficacy.[6-8]

In addition to imbalanced mainstream reporting, social media has played a role in discouraging HPV vaccine use, prompting numerous researchers to examine the effect of social media on public opinion. A 2017 article mapping social media exposure to HPV vaccine coverage found lower rates of coverage in states whose residents were more likely to read tweets about conspiracy theories and safety concerns. This study noted that positive tweets about the HPV vaccine were twice as common as negative ones, but that negative tweets were retweeted with twice the frequency.[9] A 2019, U.S.-based, systematic review of forty-four articles on the role of social media on HPV vaccination found that the World Wide Web improved public awareness and knowledge of the HPV vaccine but didn't encourage greater uptake.[10]

A different U.S.-based study in 2019 attributed 60 percent of social media users' decision-making to the influence of the posts they read, noting social media users were more likely to remember so-called HPV vaccine harms than benefits. Investigators concluded that most anti-vax sentiment among social media users arose from questions related to HPV vaccine safety and efficacy,[11] and that negative posts attracted more attention than favorable ones.[12] In other words, once the anti-vax outlook picks up steam on social media, it appears to propel the public's imagination like a runaway train.

Good Information – and Lots of It

Countering misinformation based on fear, suspicion, and sensationalist reporting requires excellent and relentless public health messaging. Governments and health care systems at all levels must not only fight bad information, but also supply good information – lots of it, all the time. This expenditure of time, money, and energy demands public and civic will built on the valuing of women's health. Nothing less than lives are at stake.

Morgan was one of those people who needed good information. An upbeat, glass-half-full dental office manager from Des Moines, Iowa, Morgan was completely unprepared when her doctor said, "Morgan, I am sorry. But you have cervical cancer." She was twenty-four. No, that isn't a typo: Morgan was diagnosed with cervical cancer at twenty-four.

Morgan received her unexpected diagnosis despite, for the most part, "doing everything right." In particular, she'd been getting screened for cervical cancer in accordance with recommended guidelines. Morgan had gone to a local Planned Parenthood clinic to have her first Pap smear at twenty-one and received "normal" test results. Three years later, in keeping with recommended screening intervals, she returned for her next Pap test, only to receive an "abnormal" result. After a follow-up and biopsies, Morgan was sent to a gynecologic oncologist on February 4, 2015. She keenly recalls the date. "I hardly remember anything he said after those three words, 'You have cancer.' I do remember the box of Kleenex in the conference room, and boy, did I use them."

I was stunned to hear the age of Morgan's diagnosis – half the average age of diagnosis at fifty – along with her cancer progression to Stage 3B. Cervical cancer this advanced at such a young age is practically unheard of. The radiation and chemotherapy treatment were aggressive and grueling, causing a series of dangerous bowel obstructions. Morgan's cancer recurred a year later, this time in her lung, but further chemotherapy gave her long-term remission. Since then, Morgan has been living cancer-free, calling herself blessed. "My doctor said only three to five percent of people with my advanced stage of cancer who suffer lung recurrence are cured," she said. "This time, I am thrilled to be 'rare.'"

None of these circumstances had to happen. Morgan was fourteen the year the HPV vaccine was introduced in the United States. Had she opted for the vaccine then, Morgan could have avoided her diagnosis altogether. Instead, she became part of the majority: the 83 percent of teens who did not receive HPV vaccination during its first year of availability – either because they were not offered the vaccine, or they opted out.

"I didn't know a whole lot about it," she recalled during our face-to-face interview. "I remember telling my mom, 'No, I don't want the vaccine.'" Then she paused, as if to consider the weight of her statement. "To this day, if you were to ask my mom, she regrets ever letting me make that decision."

Morgan blames neither her mom nor herself for refusing a vaccine 99 percent effective in preventing the HPV-16 strain. "I don't think I quite understood the connection between HPV and cancer and the vaccine." Morgan shook her head ever so slightly, looking away. "And, well," she continued ruefully, "I said those famous last words about cancer that all people say: 'That'll never happen.' And then ten years later, it happened. It happened to me: HPV-16. My cancer was caused by HPV-16!"

We were both silent. It felt like a moment of silence to acknowledge a death: the death of her fertility, the death of her normal bladder and bowel function, the death of what she called her "lightness of being" – all, now, irreversibly gone, while Morgan was still not yet thirty. And while she has moved forward, a testament to her resilience, I pondered just how different Morgan's life could have been with a robust public health campaign. Had there simply been good information.

"Yes," Morgan agreed, "I now *love* telling everyone I can just how important it is to get this vaccine."

Morgan is not unusual in her choice to opt out. According to national immunization survey data from the U.S. Centers for Disease Control and Prevention, only 17 percent of girls aged thirteen to fifteen were being vaccinated against cervical cancer in 2008, a year after Morgan was offered the vaccine. Seventeen percent represents a strikingly low initial uptake compared even with a country like Japan, despite Japan's subsequent reversal. While the number of American girls in the target age range for full vaccination has gradually increased – about 55 percent of them were getting vaccinated by 2020 – the United States still lags significantly behind other countries of similar income levels, including England, Australia, Spain, Scotland, and Switzerland (Figure 10.1). And a lot of that reluctance can be explained by looking at people's hang-ups about sex.

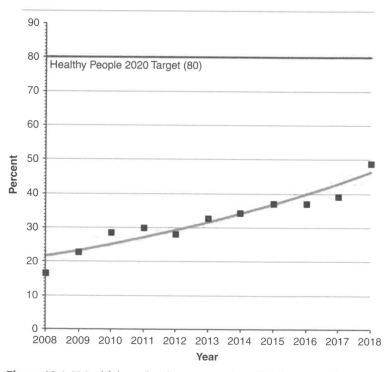

Bar graph showing U.S. girls' vaccination rates against HPV by age and year, 2008–2018.

Figure 10.1 U.S. girls' vaccination rates against HPV by age and year
Source: "HPV Vaccination." (April 2022). Accessed Jan 29, 2023. https://progressreport.cancer.gov/prevention/hpv_immunization.

You Can't Take the Sex Out of "Sexually Transmitted"

There's no getting around the fact that HPV is sexually transmitted, and that cervical cancer happens to be a "below-the-belt" disease involving females and female reproductive systems. When those medical facts meet the formidable obstacle of sexual stigma, they invite social, cultural, and religious perspectives that dramatically inhibit vaccine acceptance.

In the years after the United States first approved the HPV vaccine, not everyone appreciated its astonishing effectiveness. The notion that a sexually transmitted infection caused cervical cancer provoked consternation among some parents and providers. The vaccine's target age range, generally far younger than the onset of sexual activity, confused and alarmed those who deemed the vaccine as an enticement for preteen and teen girls to have sex. Despite multiple worldwide studies demonstrating that vaccination has little influence on when preteens or teens have sex – and peer-reviewed research trials showing no definitive link to risky sexual behaviors – the HPV vaccine has become a lightning rod for conservative religious organizations.[13-15]

Among those weighing in is Focus on the Family, an evangelical, parachurch, policy-and-media giant whose socially and politically conservative values garnered them $100 million USD from supporters and customers in 2020 alone.[16] Although Focus on the Family endorsed the vaccine in 2019,[17] twelve years earlier, in 2007, the group was promoting chastity, stating that "above any available health intervention – abstinence until marriage and faithfulness after marriage is the best and primary practice in preventing HPV and other STIs."[18] The organization's continued unwillingness to endorse universal HPV vaccine use undermined uptake of the vaccine among their many followers.

The Rome-based Catholic Medical Association weighed in on the controversy as well, with what felt like a wet blanket of mixed messages to those working toward getting lifesaving shots in arms. While acknowledging the HPV vaccine had some value, the CMA simultaneously touted the importance of chastity for preventing sexually transmitted infections. It offered this anodyne endorsement: "Healing and preventing diseases, no matter what their source, are acts of mercy and a moral good. The fact that HPV is spread primarily by sexual contact does not render vaccination against it unethical."[19]

I'm familiar with parental and social anxiety around children's emerging sexuality. As a parent of two boys (now men) and in my work as a gynecologist, I know that talking about sex with kids can be uncomfortable, even triggering. The recommended age range for maximum efficacy of the HPV vaccine demands that many of us talk about sex with our children before we probably want to. This stressful moment alone can certainly lead many parents to opt out altogether as a matter of simple avoidance – just another reason why robust, relentless public health messaging, including how-to-talk-to-your-child scripts for parents, is essential for acceptance of this lifesaving vaccine.

In the arena of sexual stigma, public health campaigns must not only account for fears around children's incipient sexuality, but the more substantial issue of fertility as well. Recommendations that solely target young women often raise suspicions in communities historically preferential to boys, and the recommended age range of nine to fourteen coincides with a time in which many girls in lower-income countries are preparing for their childbearing years. Rumors of covert contraception or sterility are easy to start and hard to combat.

The notion that a vaccine might lead to infertility is not a new one; even the polio vaccine – which saved countless cases of paralysis and lives since its invention in the 1950s – has been accused of causing infertility.[20] Not surprisingly, the HPV vaccine has been swept up in these baseless claims. In a small trial between 2009 and 2014, scientists in France studied perceptions of the HPV vaccine as it was introduced to twenty-nine lower-income countries and indeed found that many communities believed it was being used to sterilize young girls.[21] Even the built-in delay between vaccination and disease prevention presents a challenge in promoting the HPV vaccine to higher- and lower-income countries alike. Vaccinating a nine-year-old to prevent cancer that may develop twenty or thirty years later seems nebulous and unappealing – unlike preventing measles or chicken pox with vaccines designed to act almost immediately after vaccination.

Taking the Show on the Road

Focus on the Family's position paper on the HPV vaccine in 2007 upheld not just their religious values, but their political ones as well. Ultimately, they came around to endorsing a vaccine to address a sexually transmitted infection. But what they couldn't, and wouldn't, bend on is how that vaccine got delivered – not in schools. This curious moment in HPV vaccine history is where sex and logistics meet the American political landscape.

Logistics – the actual delivery of a vaccine to a body – is the unrecognized, unglamorous workhorse of the immunization world. Developing a vaccine can win you a Nobel Prize. Funding and financing it is the job of politicians and powerbrokers. Promoting it and administering it is the purview of public health officials and physicians with their titles and campaigns. But crafting a plan to actually move vaccines from the manufacturer around the world is the real feat: trucks, refrigerators, information tracing, venues, staffing. All of these factors present a particular challenge for a vaccine whose target age range does not match established immunization protocols for infants and children. Many countries have systems for administering vaccines against polio, measles, mumps, rubella, and diphtheria. But every country has had to create new logistical infrastructure for the delivery of the HPV vaccine to its preteen and teenage children. That infrastructure is so important, in fact, that lowest-income countries must be able to provide a detailed vaccine delivery and administration plan before being considered for Gavi funding.

To address these infrastructure challenges, many higher- and lower-income countries administer the HPV vaccine in schools. School-based vaccination is a remarkably efficient system. An evaluation of school-based delivery models for immunization in England between 2015 and 2016 found that more than 85 percent of children received two doses of the HPV vaccine at around fourteen.[22] In 2015, Australia demonstrated a similar uptake via school-based delivery, with almost 78 percent of their girls receiving their recommended dosage at fifteen. A 2016 *Pediatrics* review of interventions to increase vaccination rates found higher participation rates in places like Scotland, Spain, and Switzerland, all of which use the school-delivery model.[23]

And yet, school-based delivery has encountered a tepid reception in a highly resourced country like the United States. In the United States, by contrast, the logistical and infrastructure choice for HPV vaccination was left to state legislatures who – faced with tremendous pushback over requiring the vaccine for school entry – never got far enough to advance the plan. One year after its U.S. introduction, forty-one out of fifty states had introduced some kind of HPV vaccine legislation. But as of July 2022, only Rhode Island, Hawaii, Virginia, Washington, D.C., and Puerto Rico required HPV vaccination for school attendance – with a parental opt-out option – and only Rhode Island, a state of just over 1 million with no local health departments, offers school delivery of the vaccine.[24,25]

The history of HPV vaccination in the United States reflects a widespread mindset. The concept of schools mandating immunizations and exchanging the authority of the home for the school is, well, un-American. Texas governor Rick Perry tried to counter this thinking in 2007 when he signed an executive order requiring all sixth-grade girls, typically eleven or twelve years old, in the state to receive the HPV vaccine. While Perry called the vaccine "an incredible opportunity to effectively target and prevent cervical cancer," the *Texas Tribune* dubbed Perry's order "one of the most controversial decisions of his more-than-10-year reign as Texas governor."[26] The state's conservative parent and religious organizations agreed, vocally opposing the order to make the HPV vaccine mandatory, which the Texas legislature duly overturned.[27]

When the media then discovered Perry's financial ties to Merck & Co., a key manufacturer of the HPV vaccine, they went wild. But when they further learned that the governor's former chief of staff was now a lobbyist for Merck and had donated $6,000 USD to his re-election campaign, the primary victim of the outcry was not Perry, but the Texas girls denied the HPV vaccine, which had become embroiled in political scandal and an ugly, emotional battle about parental rights and sexual liberty.

A decade and a half later, researchers in Texas did evaluate the uptake of school-based vaccination in the Rio Grande Valley, an area Chapters 8 and 10 identified as having scant cervical cancer screening, and thus one for whom many would find HPV vaccination the only prevention option. Although students in three Rio Grande Valley schools learned about the benefits of HPV vaccination, just one school, Veterans Middle School, hosted a school-based, on-site vaccination program. The study found that students who received both the education and on-site vaccination programming were more than 3.6 times likelier to get vaccinated than students attending schools only promoting the HPV vaccine. Although the Rio Grande school's enthusiasm for the vaccine represents a U.S. anomaly, it confirms the advantage of school-based vaccination for boosting HPV vaccine uptake.[*]

Despite the clear benefits of vaccinating kids in schools, the idea has never really taken off in the United States. With rare exceptions like the Rio Grande Valley program, the United States continues to rely on a clinic-based delivery model to

---

[*] This study involved more than 2,000 middle-school students enrolled in three different schools in the Rio Grande City Consolidated Independent School District. Physician-led education on HPV and HPV vaccines was provided for parents/guardians, school nurses/staff, and pediatric/family medicine providers in the surrounding community. S. Kaul, T. Q. N. Do, E. Hsu, *et al.*, "School-Based Human Papillomavirus Vaccination Program for Increasing Vaccine Uptake in an Underserved Area in Texas," *Papillomavirus Res* **8** (Dec 2019): 100189. https://doi.org/10.1016/j.pvr.2019.100189 www.ncbi.nlm.nih.gov/pubmed/31654772

offer first-level prevention against cervical cancer. This model requires individual practitioners and parents to be informed and act with agency, two precarious assumptions that bring us right back to what's been missing – the need for aggressive and widespread public health campaigns: once again, "good information."

Denmark's Formidable "Information Army"

The obstacles against universal uptake of the HPV vaccine that arise from misinformation provoked by fear, rumors, sexual stigma, and political battles can make the WHO's commitment to eliminate cervical cancer by 2030 sound like pie-in-the-sky thinking. The magic bullet of the HPV vaccine – a shot that stops a cancer – needs an army of public health officials with a battle plan accounting for every foe, including disinformation. Denmark built such an army.

The HPV vaccine was introduced into Denmark's routine vaccination schedule in 2009 and quickly reached an astonishing 90 percent uptake among twelve-year-old girls. But in 2014, after reports of post-immunization pain and fatigue circulated in the media, that rate dropped to 40 percent, prompting understandable alarm by the Danish Health Authority.

Denmark health officials began their counterattack by opening an investigation into why parents were opting out of vaccinating their daughters. They rooted out the national news media as the primary source of stories about unfounded vaccine dangers. With this information, the Danish Health Authority began coalition building, and, in 2017, in concert with the Danish Cancer Society and the Danish Medical Association, they launched an information campaign called "Stop HPV, Stop Cervical Cancer." This influential group of allies pitched favorable articles about the vaccine and cervical cancer prevention to newspapers and lifestyle magazines and started a Facebook page encouraging people to ask questions and share stories about the vaccine and cervical cancer. Within just nine months, this robust effort yielded results: twice as many girls – nearly 31,000 – opted for the vaccine compared with just 15,000 the year before.

Danish investigators have actually been able to pinpoint July 2013 as the country's low point for vaccination uptake, which coincided with a verified increase in Google searches for "HPV side effects" and negative vaccine media coverage. Figure 10.2 shows both the damaging effect of negative news coverage and the successful impact of the public health response on vaccine acceptance in Denmark.

The Denmark story makes clear that every HPV vaccination campaign, no matter how successful, is subject to fear, suspicion, and false reports. Research from the University of North Carolina at Chapel Hill shows that despite rebounding vaccination rates, about 26,000 Danish girls remain unvaccinated as a result of misinformation.[28] Lives at risk yet again for want of that aforementioned good information.

But unlike Japan, which suffered more than a decade of no HPV vaccinations at all, Denmark battled back quickly, responding with curiosity, fact-finding, coalition building, and a powerful public health campaign that included wise use of

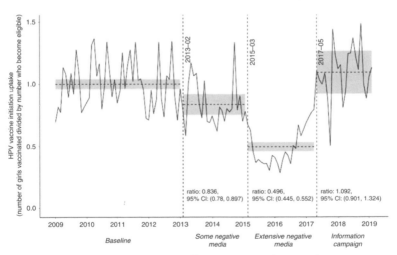

Figure 10.2 Effects of negative media on HPV vaccine uptake
Source: Hansen, P. R., M. Schmidtblaicher, and N. T. Brewer. "Resilience of HPV Vaccine Uptake in Denmark: Decline and Recovery." *Vaccine* 38, no. 7 (Feb 11, 2020): 1842–48. https://doi.org/10.1016/j.vaccine.2019.12.019
https://www.ncbi.nlm.nih.gov/pubmed/31918860

social media. The Danish experience makes clear that to succeed, HPV vaccination programs must include communication
plans that anticipate possible objections and disinformation at
local, regional, and national levels.

The fight to end cervical cancer is clearly an all-hands-on-deck
fight. In addition to the obvious obstacles of vaccine cost and
supply, we face the foes of sex, lies, and logistics: fights that
demand time, money, and human energy. When those oppon-
ents get the best of us, as they did in Japan, Texas, and temporarily in Denmark – and in countless other places around the
world – we must learn with curiosity, find allies, and counterattack with relentless good information. Nothing less than lives
are at stake.

11 PUTTING OUT THE FIRES: OBSTACLES TO SCREENING

Most of us have smoke alarms in our homes. We sleep better knowing these handy little gadgets are armed for the first sign of fire. That's because smoke alarms work: in the United States, their use rose from 10 percent in 1975 to a whopping 95 percent by 2000, and, because they're commonplace, we've seen the number of home-fire deaths cut in half.[1] These simple, inexpensive devices have been hailed as "the greatest success story in fire safety."[2,3] Success, indeed.

But smoke alarms don't put out fires; they just tell us that one exists. Preventing fire damage relies on countless variables: a working battery in the alarm, someone home to hear the alarm, a working telephone to alert the fire department, firefighters on duty, trucks and firefighting equipment, working water supply lines. Putting out a fire is a complicated venture. So is screening for cervical cancer. Complicated, yes – but a reliable means of saving lives.

A cervical screening test, like a smoke alarm, is health care's first line of defense against cervical cancer – and it's profoundly effective. Consistent, widespread use of the Pap smear has cut U.S. cervical cancer rates in half over the past thirty years. Globally, hundreds of thousands of lives have been saved through large-scale efforts to find and treat cervical cancer and the pre-cancers that cause it.

And while the HPV vaccine will save hundreds of thousands of future cervical cancer cases, for generations of persons with cervixes born too early to benefit from the vaccine, for those without access to it, and for the very small percentage of cancers the vaccine does not stop,[*] cervical cancer screening is the only way to put out the fires of cancer that continue to disfigure and destroy.

Those Fires Are Raging

In 2015, researchers in Malawi[4] surveyed established national cancer plans in several African countries and found that, despite guidelines advising women to get screened for cervical cancer, the actual number who did so came to less than 5 percent. A 2020 review of nineteen studies over five years of cervical cancer screening in sub-Saharan Africa showed screening rates ranging from little more than half of eligible women to none at all.[5] According to a 2017 study, less than 10 percent of women in many lower-income Asian countries have received cervical cancer screening. [6]

Not a Fire: A Conflagration

Even in higher-income countries, where cervical screening is relatively more available, cervical cancer hotspots erupt, "burning" women who are largely poor, not White, rural, marginalized, or Indigenous. In Australia, the country most on track to eliminate cervical cancer, screening rates are far lower for Aboriginal rather than non-Aboriginal women.[7,8] In the United Kingdom, 30 percent of women are not screened for cervical cancer – despite the fact that it's free! Researchers there have discovered the limitations of publicly funded screening appointments. Without childcare or support systems enabling working women to attend a clinic's twice-monthly screening days, these important appointments are forsaken altogether. Data from a 2019 National Center for Health Statistics survey showed that

---

[*] The bivalent and quadrivalent HPV vaccines prevent 70 percent of cervical cancer caused by HPV-virus types and the nonavalent HPV vaccine prevents 90 percent of cervical cancer caused by HPV-virus types. N. Van de Velde, M. C. Boily, M. Drolet, *et al.*, "Population-Level Impact of the Bivalent, Quadrivalent, and Nonavalent Human Papillomavirus Vaccines: A Model-Based Analysis," *J Natl Cancer Inst* **104**, no. 22 (Nov 21 2012): 1712–23. https://doi.org/10.1093/jnci/djs395 www.ncbi.nlm.nih.gov/pubmed/23104323

while 74 percent of U.S. women twenty-one to sixty-five were up to date with cervical screening, national screening levels diminished in proportion to education and income levels. U.S. screening rates were as low as 59 percent among persons with cervixes who had less than a high school education. Only 64 percent of women with incomes less than twice the national poverty level – or roughly $50,000 USD a year for a family of four – are getting screened.[9] As discussed in Chapter 8, some parts of the United States, such as the Rio Grande Valley in Texas, have screening rates as low as 15 percent. The United States and other higher-income countries inexcusably account for plenty of those cervical cancer screening–avoidant hotspots.

These figures represent just a fraction of a dismal global picture, where 90 percent of women dying of cervical cancer come from countries with little to no access to screening. Why is there not enough for these women? What is preventing us from quenching this inferno for good?

Like smoke alarms, cervical screening tests depend on multiple, interconnected factors to successfully sound the alarm. These factors include trained providers, infrastructure, equipment, accessibility to services, data monitoring, and system evaluation. Screening efficacy is additionally affected by cultural stigma, systemic bias, and (always) the rock-bottom question: *What is a woman worth?* Of course, money plays a key role in improving the "cervical cancer alarm system" worldwide and ensuring women's protection against cervical cancer is a top priority – just as is saving a home from a fire.

The Smoke Alarms of Cervical Cancer Prevention

Cervical cancer screening starts with one of three tests: HPV-DNA testing, the Pap smear, or a Visual Inspection with Acetic Acid (VIA) test. Of the three, an HPV-DNA test is most sensitive to detecting abnormalities. In 2020, the American Cancer Society recommended HPV-DNA testing in the United States for all persons with cervixes.[10] The World Health Organization's latest screening guidelines (developed by the WHO steering committee, of which I was a member) set the standards for delivery of cervical cancer prevention services; they recommend HPV-DNA testing when feasible. While many lower-income countries would love the option of HPV-DNA testing, no affordable and effective HPV-DNA tests are available for cash-strapped countries like Malawi or Kenya, or Cambodia or Haiti, for that matter. Private companies, universities, and global health development groups are all working hard to develop a low-cost HPV-DNA test. But governments and global development agencies still find widespread HPV-DNA testing prohibitively expensive.

The United States now relies on HPV-DNA testing, with Pap smear testing following a positive HPV-DNA test or as a complementary measure. HPV-DNA testing is also used in other higher-income countries that can afford it. Most lower-income country guidelines, however, depend on VIA, the least expensive, most readily available screening option. VIA also happens to be the least reliable method – partly because it relies on human inspection. Its accuracy in detecting pre-cancer or cancer ranges between 40 and 70 percent. Inflammation from an infection can look like cancer, for instance, making it difficult for VIA providers to accurately assess common conditions like cervical infections or vaginal yeast infections. But VIA's well-known limitations are currently offset by its vastly greater affordability for nations confronting inadequate or close-to-nonexistent health care budgets. VIA tests are like smoke alarms that work half to three-quarters of the time at best: better than nothing at all, but not great.[11]

"Firefighters Wanted": Prevention Demands Personnel

For lower-income countries trying to establish and maintain cervical cancer screening programs, trained health care providers are another critical resource in scant supply. In 2017, researchers in Kenya found that just 3.5 percent of eligible women were being screened for cervical cancer,[12] and a subsequent study identified the culprit as an insufficient number of trained health care workers. They pointed to a physician-to-population ratio ranging from 1:21,000 in a community with three hospitals to a shocking 1:143,000 in a rural community.[13] (To put it in perspective, higher-income countries report ratios of medical providers to people somewhere between 195:100,000 and 500:100,000.)* In other words, the search for a provider among persons with cervixes in Kenya can look like going into a crowded football stadium, sitting in the stands, and hoping to meet the star player. The odds of being able to secure that medical provider are so discouraging that it's easy to see why a woman would give up on the very idea of getting herself screened.

Once identified and hired, health care workers still require the necessary skills. Training providers to perform tests like the Pap or the VIA requires significant, sustained investment that often exacts a toll on other health programming. It takes five to ten days to train a provider to perform a VIA test. In countries where clinics often have a single provider, this five- to ten-day absence for training precludes a provider from seeing patients, leading to clinic closures or restrictions.

In addition, VIA providers need to maintain or improve their skills, which requires a system of "supportive supervision." Supervisors must monitor trainees in person or digitally, such

---

* To put the lower-income country's plight in perspective, in higher-income countries documenting access to health care providers, the number of active physicians per 100,000 people is at least 25 times higher. A 2022 U.S. state-by-state review by the Becker Hospital Review group found that the number of U.S. physicians per 100,000 people ranged from a high of 466 in Massachusetts to 285 in Washington State (where I practice medicine) to 211 in Wyoming (where I grew up, a relatively rural, sparsely populated state), with the lowest of the fifty states being Idaho, offering a ratio of 196 to 100,000. www.beckershospitalreview.com/workforce/this-state-has-the-most-physicians-per-capita.html, accessed Jan 20, 2023.
These figures were similar in higher-income countries outside the United States. A 2017 study published in the *British Medical Journal* evaluating access to physicians in Europe found that the lowest physician-to-population ratios were in the United Kingdom, with 280 doctors for every 100,000 people, while the average across 33 European countries was 300 physicians. Specifically, Austria was among the highest, with 510 doctors for every 100,000 people. Germany, Italy, Lithuania, Norway, and Switzerland all had more than 400 doctors for every 100,000 people (*BMJ* 2017;**357**: j2940).
While the ratio of providers to patients in these higher-income countries does vary markedly, all higher-income countries have roughly 100 times the number of providers per patient as does Kenya.

as using shared images via cell phone. This means covering supervisors' travel or technology costs. For countries with already-stressed human capital demands, obtaining and retaining this level of supervision poses yet another challenge, and one not all are in a position to tackle.

Provider shortages such as these are not the burden of lower-income countries alone. In the context of cervical cancer, insufficient medical personnel can discourage patients in higher-income countries from getting screened – the reduced supply of experts driving up costs. Human Rights Watch reports assessing cervical cancer prevention in southern U.S. states like Alabama[14] and Georgia[15] cite the difficulty for lower-income residents in finding affordable screening tests or follow-up colposcopies and biopsies. In these southern states – and particularly among rural residents – the shortage of trained gynecologists or even gynecologists offering services on a sliding scale gets in the way of significant efforts to prevent cervical cancer.

Bikes, Buses, and Rutted Roads: Physical Hurdles to Health Care

Finding a health care provider is just as challenging as getting to that provider. With more clinics found in urban settings, women in rural or remote areas seeking cervical cancer screening – whether they live in lower- or higher-income countries – can find the lack of transportation or distance to and from a clinic difficult enough to stop them in their tracks.

Australia offers publicly funded cervical cancer care to all of its citizens, but that doesn't come with a ride to the clinic for primarily Indigenous women living in the interior of the country struggling to access care hundreds of miles away. The same problem holds true for Canadian women living in the rugged, sparsely populated Northwest Territories, or for American women living in the interior of Alaska, where no roads exist, and settlements must be reached by small airplanes. In the state of Alabama, no public transportation is available to carry a woman three hours[14] to one of the few clinics caring for lower-income women; the roads exist, but for many of these women, hiring a ride to such a distant destination is just too expensive. Inevitably, this absence of access means that women who are poor, of color, or Indigenous are likely to miss out on screening. In countries like Haiti or Sudan, where significantly fewer people own a car or even a motorcycle or bicycle, a woman must either walk or depend on public transit – the latter of which is often decades-old, held together with rebuilt parts, unreliable, and requiring money to ride.

The bottom line is that a woman needs a form of transport to get to her screening appointments, which in turn requires a passable road system. Yet, transportation networks in lower-income countries often present another barrier when roads are treacherous or even impassable, depending on whether routes to clinics require crossings through mountains or deserts, or are heavily affected by seasonal weather patterns.

I have encountered these problems firsthand in my work in Nicaragua, Liberia, Kenya, and Malawi. I recall traveling with my colleague Dr. Lameck Chinula to work in a rural clinic in Malawi and spending one hour covering twenty kilometers of road due to the ruts, bumps, washouts, curves, and animal crossings. One time, we sat for fifteen minutes waiting for a herd of cattle to meander across the road. We were spared only by the fact that it was dry season, allowing us to eventually reach the clinic. In wet season, the clinic would have been unreachable by road, leaving women in need of cervical cancer screening services out of luck for up to half a year. *Half a year!*

Garbage Bags, Cell Phones, and a Twenty-Five-Dollar Piece of Metal

If and when a woman finally does reach a health care clinic, she can encounter one wanting for the most basic equipment. Speculums, the piece of equipment that holds the vaginal

walls out of the way for a closer look at the cervix, cost about
$5 USD apiece for the plastic version and $25 USD for the metal
ones.[16] At Harborview Hospital clinic in Seattle, we have drawers and drawers of equipment regularly cleaned and ready for
use, including (typically metal) speculums of different sizes. But
a clinic in a lower-income country typically owns just a few
speculums. The more expensive, but durable metal speculums
require special disinfectants and personnel to clean them after
use. Plastic speculums are disposable, single-use items in the
United States, but in lower-income clinics where I've worked,
I have seen them cleaned and reused multiple times. When
I worked in Nicaragua, we scheduled just two women a day for
screening, because the clinic possessed two metal speculums
that could only be cleaned at the end of the day. When I visited
a busy urban clinic in Namibia, the providers could only perform gynecological examinations on Tuesday afternoons when
the clinic could provide clean speculums. In both Nicaragua and
Namibia, a trained provider was available, but women went
without screening for lack of a $5 to $25 USD piece of plastic
or metal.

Medical equipment we take for granted in privileged settings
is persistently in short supply in lower-income countries. At the
Lilongwe clinic in Malawi, we used plastic garbage bags to cover
examination tables, and patients knew in advance to bring their
own cloths or blankets to cover themselves. Even lighting presents a challenge in lower-income countries, where rural citizens may not have electricity, and urban areas experience
intermittent delays and shortages. My colleague Dr. Chinula
regularly uses the flashlight feature on his cell phone to properly visualize a cervix – a built-in problem when the phone loses
battery life and needs to be recharged.

If it's this difficult to provide basics like speculums and lighting for accurate cervical screenings – not to mention the trained
health care providers who know how to use them – it's not hard
to imagine the challenges to every subsequent step: biopsy
taking and reading, and follow-up treatment. Which leads me
to a grim reality for women around the world: cervical

screening is pointless without proper evaluation and treatment of suspicious findings. We can screen every cervix in the world, but unless we can provide follow-up care, we're not going to catch cervical cancer soon enough to save a life. It's like smoke alarms blaring with no one there to put out the fire.

Blaring Alarms and No One's Home: Why Follow-Up Is Vital

Screening alone will not save lives. Screening – followed by necessary treatment for pre-cancer – is the magical formula for preventing cancer and death. When screening identifies pre-cancer, it must be treated with ablation or excision. And when a provider sees suspicious signs of possible cancer, that cervix needs to be biopsied to confirm cancer. Think about the persons with cervixes who somehow overcome the problems of scarce clinics, shortages of providers, limited testing, lack of transportation, and insufficient access to tests. They'll likely face that gauntlet a second time as they seek follow-up treatment for suspicious findings. Where providers, access, and equipment are already scarce, follow-up treatment can be abysmal to nonexistent.

My Kenyan colleague Dr. Nelly Mugo sees the deadly disconnect between screening tests and follow-up treatment. When I spoke with her in 2020, she pointed out that only about 20 percent of Kenyan women who screened positive for cervical pre-cancer using VIA were actually receiving cryotherapy treatment, a common way to remove pre-cancerous cells by freezing them with carbon dioxide or liquid nitrogen. Obtaining those gases can be difficult and costly, meaning that women diagnosed with treatable cervical pre-cancer in Kenya – or any country where basic equipment is unavailable – will be denied treatment for want of a gas. When I spoke with Dr. Mugo again in 2022, she told me that Kenya was switching to thermal ablation for treatment and had deemed the improvement of cervical cancer treatment rates a high priority. Still, imagine this: Kenyan women testing positive for cervical pre-cancer or cancer and receiving only the knowledge they need treatment – along with the realization they won't be able to get it.

Low-income women or women living in rural areas of higher-income countries can end up in the same heart-sinking predicament. Follow-up care for cervical cancer often involves an array of specialists, specialized equipment, and a series of expensive and onerous clinic appointments that simply render lifesaving care out of reach.

Taboo, Stigma, and Systemic Bias: Prevention Roadblocks

Public health messaging is an important part of any screening program; it educates citizens and normalizes a health message over time. Communication in support of cervical screening must allow women to become used to the idea of having their bodies on display. Few other medical procedures require undressing, dangling one's legs in stirrups while spreading knees apart, and allowing a health care provider – sometimes a stranger – to do an examination. In some countries, even the idea of such an exam is unthinkable. "Women do not discuss their private parts," said Dr. Mugo, nonetheless a fierce proponent of spreading the word about screening. "[Advocates for cervical cancer screening] need to get beyond medical people and talk to the general population – both women and men – about cervical cancer."

My colleague in Malawi, Dr. Abiba Ngwira, who served there as head of Monitoring and Evaluation for the International Training and Education Center for Health, is similarly concerned about promoting cervical screening in her country. "Women just do not talk about the vagina or cervical cancer." Taboos around female anatomy, she said, present a universal challenge for prevention messaging.

Fundamental taboos about sex make talking about a sexually transmitted viral cancer doubly challenging. The stigma associated with HPV turned out to be a common theme among everyone I spoke with for this book. An "HPV-positive" label can present a psychological obstacle to screening by implying how often or with whom someone has had sex – despite the majority of sexually active adults contracting HPV infections in their lifetimes.

In 2020, a study by UK-based advocacy group Jo's Cervical Cancer Trust tried to quantify the stigma of an HPV diagnosis.[17] One-third of the 2,000 local women interviewed considered HPV a taboo topic, and 39 percent would not want anyone to know they had HPV. Forty percent said an HPV diagnosis would negatively affect their dating lives, and 43 percent said it would adversely affect their sex lives. Half of the respondents would consider ending a relationship with someone who had HPV. The results show the chilling effect of cultural shame and fear of an HPV diagnosis on cervical cancer prevention via screening.

For women who live in countries or regions with high rates of HIV, like sub-Saharan Africa, cervical screening is often offered in tandem with HIV care, an efficient use of resources given HIV's accelerant effect on HPV. But attending an HIV clinic is a source of embarrassment for many women; that stigma can deter women without HIV from accessing screening.

Effective communication about cervical screening must do more to help women overcome natural aversions to the procedure, while remaining aware of underlying cultural taboos and stigma. Public health messaging needs to be culturally and contextually specific, taking into account diverse beliefs and practices. A 2016 Canadian systematic review evaluating literature on barriers to cancer screening among South Asian immigrants in Canada, the United Kingdom, and the United States confirmed this finding. Lower screening rates among these groups were attributed to a lack of targeted messaging.[18] Alternatively, researchers suggested communicating with this group by incorporating their family-based, holistic approach to medical care, while considering their overall lack of familiarity with preventative medicine and with cervical cancer screening in particular.

Studies about screening promotion for Indigenous people in North America and New Zealand – known to have lower screening rates than other ethnic groups in those countries – stress a similar need for tailored communication campaigns.[19,20]

I came face-to-face with the challenges of culturally sensitive messaging in 2008 while attending a medical meeting on forensic medicine in Istanbul. During the meeting, I gave a teaching lecture on speculum use for pelvic examinations. I was shocked when both male and female health care providers in the audience told me that speculum use was viewed as a threat for ending a woman's virginity. In Turkey, they told me, a woman whose chastity is called into question may have trouble securing a husband or be subjected to socially condoned violence from her husband and family. Imagine trying to craft a positive message about cervical cancer screening to Turkish women when the means of prevention could potentially be perceived as more threatening than the cancer itself.

At Harborview's obstetrics and gynecology clinic where I work in Seattle, we try our best to accommodate patients whose religious beliefs run counter to receiving pelvic exams from male medical providers. But sometimes a female provider simply isn't available. Patients whose wishes can't be accommodated can fall behind on their cervical cancer prevention regimens. These outcomes are always a concern, both at our clinic and elsewhere. Many clinics have even fewer female medical providers, and sometimes a patient may choose between staying up to date with her screening appointments or temporarily setting aside cherished beliefs – an experience that might be distressing and even traumatizing – in order to undergo an examination from the only available provider who happens to be male.

Deep-rooted cultural objections to the standard Westernized approach to screening – whether they're about the screening process itself or who provides it – reflect the range of attitudes and fears that get in the way of women combating cervical cancer. These differing philosophies are a reminder to promote cervical screening with more than a one-size-fits-all message.

What's more, culturally and contextually specific messaging must acknowledge systemic racism as an obstacle to screening. Both conscious discrimination and unconscious bias can affect the quality of the examination a woman receives. Teolita, the Black woman described in Chapter 3 who died of cervical cancer in her thirties, had gone to the emergency room with abnormal bleeding twice in three months, but never received a pelvic examination in the emergency room. By the time she saw a gynecologist, she had Stage 4 cervical cancer, a finding ordinarily picked up during a routine pelvic exam. Researchers in the United States and in the United Kingdom have found that regardless of racial biases being conscious or unconscious, they interfere with women's access to care or the effectiveness of the care itself.

In 2020, researchers at Tuskegee University in Alabama[21] compared state differences between Black and White women in cervical cancer diagnosis, treatment, and survival. Their findings – which hold implications for Teolita's experience – were consistent with national data: 2,124 cervical cancer cases in Alabama between 2004 and 2013 confirmed that Black women were diagnosed with more advanced cervical cancer and thus less likely to survive. The study's authors attributed Black women's inequitable experience to a lack of insurance coverage and an inability to access timely screening and treatment for pre-cancer, a problem worsened for Black women living in rural Alabama. Similar findings were uncovered a year later, in 2021, in a Michigan-based study that relied on U.S. survey data of more than 7,500 women.[22] While Michigan researchers cited similar cervical cancer screening rates for Black and White women, they found Black women less likely to be informed about abnormal Pap test results and less likely to receive follow-up. In order to overcome these disparities, the authors concluded, individual U.S. states would need to overhaul existing tracking and delivery systems for cervical cancer screening results, sponsor culturally appropriate messages about the significance of results and follow-up, and develop a means for consistent follow-up and pre-cancer treatment.

In support of these findings, recent Human Rights Watch reports from Alabama and Georgia attributed higher cervical cancer rates among Black women to challenges in obtaining pre-cancer follow-up and treatment. These reports highlighted deficiencies in the "Black belt" of Alabama and Georgia that included a lack of trained gynecologists to oversee abnormal screening results and the financial burdens and lack of transportation options for follow-up treatment. Once again, Black women in rural areas or without medical insurance faced the biggest hurdles to care.

Together, these studies and reports reinforce the insufficiency of single screening appointments: screening tests without follow-up are smoke alarms without emergency responders. They help explain why – in the absence of an adequate response system for screening results – more Black women are developing cervical cancer at a more advanced stage. These findings raise uncomfortable questions about the effects of racial bias on cervical cancer screening and care. Like every other obstacle, racism must be identified, rooted out, and overcome – a daunting but necessary step in preventing cervical cancer for persons with cervixes of any race.

In addition to the hurdles associated with racial bias, patients must contend with another potential source of prejudice: gender bias. Not all persons born with cervixes are women. Transgender men or gender nonbinary patients are understandably reluctant to receive pelvic exams and can face extraordinary obstacles in female-focused environments, including the dysphoria of registering for an examination at a "women's clinic." In a 2020 U.S.-based study of twenty transgender men, researchers revealed a host of barriers preventing this group from getting regularly screened, including previous negative experiences with medical clinics, low income levels, and issues related to gender identity. The study's findings reflect similar barriers in countries that typically pay for citizens' medical care. In the United Kingdom, for instance, the National Health Service only sends out reminder notices for cervical cancer screening to patients registered as female.

A 2020 Canadian-based summary of fifteen research studies about rates of and barriers to cervical cancer screening among transgender men noted that most of the respondents found a Pap test "overwhelmingly challenging, emotionally and psychologically, deterring them from screening."[23] According to research findings, the unique challenges in caring for transgender men can include anxiety arising from having an examination designed for female genital organs, like a cervix. Transgender men can also experience physical discomfort during a pelvic examination, because they typically have smaller vaginas – a common side effect of receiving testosterone treatment. The fact that many health care providers remain unfamiliar with and reticent about providing cervical cancer screening to transgender males poses a significant obstacle to their deserved and critical care.

Addressing these deterrents to care means changing individual and systemic attitudes. "Signing up for a pelvic examination is pretty awful when I don't identify as a woman," said Bailey, one of my gender nonbinary patients, "and then it only makes it worse having twenty minutes of questions about my health history asked in a way that assumes I am identifying as a female." A 2019 Canadian study of cervical cancer screening at a primary health care practice that serves 45,000 residents of Toronto found that transgender persons with cervixes were 60 percent less likely than their cisgender counterparts to have cervical screening.[24]

Jess, a forty-one-year-old therapist who lives with her wife in Berthoud, Colorado, and identifies as gender nonbinary, spoke directly to the problem of inherent bias toward heteronormative patients. Jess was just thirty-three when she was diagnosed with cervical cancer. While she'd generally kept up to date with her Pap smears every three years, a single delay in screening – one she attributed to her dread of going for the examination – resulted in a cervical cancer diagnosis, and all the attendant suffering and struggle that went along with treatment thereafter.

She described putting off her screening appointments because she was afraid of being judged for her sexual orientation. "This did not set me up to be comfortable with many gynecologists," she said, claiming the screening appointments tended to be designed for heterosexual patients. "They asked off-putting questions – and it is an off-putting, vulnerable test."

In my experience as a gynecologist providing cervical screening for persons with cervixes, I commonly hear that being "comfortable" with the person offering the pelvic examination is what patients value most, regardless of their gender or sexual orientation (Figure 11.1). All of us want to be asked questions about our health in a way that's respectful and doesn't provoke shame or make us feel judged. In the context of cervical cancer prevention, the need for sensitivity in exam rooms is even more critical for those who don't identify as heterosexual or even as women.

Acknowledging and overcoming deeply rooted, systemic biases like these, both big and small, will require a significant shift in thinking among the medical community. Until that happens, we cannot be surprised that our transgender men and gender nonbinary patients with cervixes report much lower screening rates than female-identifying patients. A cervix is a cervix. And a cervix needs care.

A cervix is a cervix. And a cervix needs care.

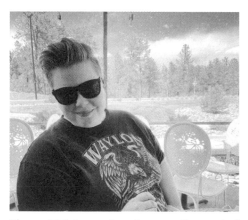

Figure 11.1 Jess, who advocates for cervical cancer screening being welcoming to all

Data: The Unsexy Hero of Cervical Screening

If the unsung hero of firefighting is the 911 dispatcher who connects frantic calls and fire stations, then the unsexy, but totally necessary hero of screening and follow-up is data collection and systems evaluation. Without centralized tracking and messaging mechanisms, countries will struggle to accurately promote current screening guidelines, count and manage screenings, follow up with those in need of further evaluation or care, justify continued funding, and even do the grim work of tabulating deaths – the latter of which can act as the catalyst to important changes in public policy.

In many lower-income countries, medical records are handwritten, hand-tabulated, and kept on paper rather than on electronic records. In Malawi, patients carry a small paper "passport" from clinic to clinic. In Namibia, the cervical cancer screening register at the clinic where I worked contained paper pages whose wide columns recorded patient information like "lives in third house behind the chicken coop on Presidential Road" and "contact village shopkeeper to get message to patient." I could imagine how challenging follow-up care would be using these rudimentary tracking and communication systems, health care provider or supply shortages aside. In countries like these, sharing information among clinicians – or through any systematic, nationwide effort – looked to me like an impossible task.

In the United States, we too lack a central tracking system for monitoring cervical cancer screening. Private insurance companies and large health systems, like my hospital clinic in Seattle, develop their own data collection and tracking systems. But the limited range of such practices, designed to service a single system and its clients, doesn't meet the robust, universal approach required to prevent and ultimately eliminate cervical cancer. Inevitably, people are overlooked: for appointments, for follow-up, even for public health messaging, which is what brings people with cervixes in for screening in the first place.

Monitoring and evaluation systems supply answers to critical questions that inform program planning: How many citizens with cervixes are being screened? How many of those screened need a follow-up biopsy or treatment for pre-cancer? Are they receiving that biopsy or treatment or not? Why? When cancer is found, how much, and at what stage? Data like these are crucial for planning the nuts and bolts of a program and making changes as needed.

In countries whose strong health guidelines are regularly reviewed and possibly changed, complex and disjointed communication systems can lead to mixed messages, missed messages, and confusion that dissuade women from screening altogether. Of course, the medical community needs to respond to new data by making timely changes to screening recommendations. But as a provider who does almost daily cervical cancer screening, I can attest that after major U.S. guideline updates in 2002, 2012, 2016, 2018, and 2020, even *I* felt confused! These changes can upset the rigor needed to enforce regular, habitual screening for cervical cancer. A 2016 study from Germany synthesized sixty-nine studies investigating barriers to new guideline adoptions and found that it typically takes "many years" for new guidelines to be broadly disseminated through national and regional regulatory bodies, professional societies, patient networks, and the general news media.[25] These are years in which – especially in the absence of strong, universal data collection, tracking, and circulation – confusion costs lives.

Politically, data are essential to reinforcing the political will and financial commitment of a country's decision-makers. Data justify the continued expense of cervical screening when those in power can say they are saving lives and quantifying the resulting return to the economy. Data tell taxpayers and budget makers alike that the expense is worth it. In the world of scarce health care dollars, data always means power. But what's also clear is that in many countries – countries as well-resourced as the United States, even – data are not offering citizens the power they should in health care, a fact that directly gets in the way of ending cervical cancer.

Scarcity Equals Suffering

By now, you will have noticed a familiar theme: "low, appallingly low, dramatically low, inadequate, absence, impoverished, less likely, scant supply, meager at best, abysmal, nonexistent." These phrases are often repeated in connection with eliminating disease on a global scale. Even though we have what we need to screen for and prevent cervical cancer, scarcity stalks us at every turn. And the cost of that scarcity is human suffering.

Ruth suffered from scarcity, and it diminished her health care in a shocking way. I met Ruth, a thirty-three-year-old mother of four, while collaborating with local health ministry officials and doctors to update Malawi's cervical cancer prevention guidelines. When I arrived at the Lilongwe gynecology clinic at 9:00 a.m. one morning, Ruth was one of forty women sitting shoulder-to-shoulder on backless, one-foot-deep benches. Ruth had traveled by bus for three hours to secure herself a place in line. When her name was called, she hurriedly tied in a handkerchief the bites of bread she carried with her as breakfast, surprised and relieved to have her name called so early.

Ruth was a small woman. Her bright yellow skirt, patterned with blue block-print, was tied around her waist, hanging halfway between her knees and flip-flops. Her headscarf, made of matching skirt fabric, was tied loosely, allowing me to see her thin and receding hair. Her vibrant clothes could not hide her deep fatigue, a kind of tiredness that one night's sleep couldn't fix. Ruth looked at least ten years older than her age. As she recounted her medical history, I understood why. I was astonished by the trials she'd endured.

Roughly one year prior to her appointment, Ruth had gone to a local primary care clinic in the town closest to her village for her first-ever VIA screening test. Her health passport contained the word *suspicious* in connection with the VIA test finding. *Suspicious* suggests possible cancer, and the patient in question is usually sent for a biopsy to confirm those findings.

But Ruth's primary clinic had neither a trained provider nor the equipment for a biopsy, much less a pathologist who could evaluate one. Based on the VIA result – the only and best test her doctor had – Ruth was told to see a cancer specialist. With no regular referral system in Malawi for patients with abnormal screening results, Ruth would have needed to find this specialist on her own.

As citizens do in countries that don't offer public or private health insurance, Ruth and her husband reached out to their extended family to pay for a specialist. Ruth managed to find an oncologist, one of the few medical doctors in Malawi who offered cancer treatment. Neither she nor her husband entirely understood her medical problem, but they knew "cancer was bad."

The oncologist proposed chemotherapy, and Ruth and her husband called on the support of a wider network of relatives to purchase the prescribed drugs for monthly infusions. The next six months of grueling treatments made Ruth's already demanding life almost impossible. Her hair fell out, and her periods stopped. She lost weight and she fought for energy just to get through each day. Ruth told me she was clear about one thing: she had to keep going. Her family needed the money from her work, and her children needed their mother.

After six punishing months of chemotherapy, the oncologist told Ruth to see a gynecologist who would examine her cervix and make sure she was cancer-free. Again, using precious family money, she got herself to a gynecologist at one of the main hospitals in the big city. There, the gynecologist could look at her cervix with a specialized microscope called a colposcope. He found no abnormalities and took a biopsy to confirm that conclusion.

Compare Ruth's trials to the typical experience of an insured or moderately well-off patient living on the U.S. West Coast and regularly going to the doctor. Patients in my Seattle clinic who undergo a cervical biopsy, for instance, usually wait three days for results, one week at the very most. Ruth waited another six months for hers.

Finally – a full year after she'd started chemotherapy – Ruth was elated to receive this welcome news: no cancer was found! The gynecologist credited Ruth's chemotherapy for curing her cancer and referred Ruth to Dr. Chinula at the main hospital in Lilongwe to be evaluated for a hysterectomy to prevent her cancer from recurring. Dr. Chinula had completed his gyne-cology training in South Africa, with additional cancer surgery training from an American gynecology oncologist. He was one of just six gynecologists in Malawi with the training needed to care for patients like Ruth, and the only one in the central Malawi geographic region. I was working with him the day Ruth arrived.

While Dr. Chinula fastened a clean, plastic trash bag on the examination table with clamps, Ruth stepped behind a cloth curtain to remove her undergarments. As she sat on the exam table, she covered her thin, atrophied legs with a cloth brought from home. Once she'd positioned her feet in the stirrups, I used the flashlight on Dr. Chinula's cell phone to provide him the necessary light for positioning the speculum in her vagina. After a few moments, he turned to me. "Would you take a look at this?" he asked. My heart sank: had he seen a big tumor or mass?

No. What Dr. Chinula and I saw was more shocking than that: Ruth's cervix was completely smooth. No irregularity, no bleed-ing, no funny color or shape. It looked healthy and completely normal. We were stunned. How could a woman, after solely receiving chemotherapy for a disease usually stopped by radi-ation and surgery, have a normal, cancer-free cervix a year later? Dr. Chinula found a colposcope in his clinic, and we looked again. Under the powerful magnification of the colpo-scope, Ruth's cervix remained clear and normal.

Dr. Chinula took a few biopsies to make sure we hadn't missed any abnormalities, and, as Ruth was putting her clothes back on, we stepped into the hallway to talk. As we pored over her health passport, we realized that no one had ever looked at Ruth's cervix between the initial "suspicious" finding and the final round of chemotherapy. Slowly, we drew a terrible conclusion.

Ruth had never had cancer.

Her whole treatment had been based on the result of the VIA, not a biopsy. Neither the provider at her primary care clinic nor the oncologist who gave her chemotherapy had done a biopsy, because they lacked the means and equipment to do one. Ruth endured six grueling months of chemotherapy and a year of living with the terrible fear she had cancer. She and her family spent desperately needed household money for treatment she didn't need – against a cancer she didn't have.

Ruth's story reflects the human costs so many women around the world face because of the phenomenon of "not enough." No trained provider for a biopsy. No equipment for a biopsy. No pathologist to read a biopsy. No insurance. Few oncologists. Distant clinics. Paltry record-keeping. I returned home from Malawi shaken by this close-up look at the consequences of screening without proper follow-up care.

It is screening – followed by necessary treatment for pre-cancer – that actually prevents cancer and death. Like a smoke alarm, a screening test alone cannot save a life. Thousands of women around the world know this all too well. Some would say Ruth was lucky, but she endured months of unnecessary, expensive, and toxic treatments. Scarcity made her suffer too.

The Role of Money in Inequity

Scarcity in health care – and cervical cancer care is no exception – often gets attributed to money: the apparent lack of "enough." Money buys equipment, trains and pays providers, builds clinics in lower-income countries. Money pays for public health messaging and data systems. But health care budgets compete with a long line of needs: national security, infrastructure, education. Even within those budgets, disparate programs jockey for their share of an already small slice of the pie.

Cervical cancer screening and treatment compete with other essentials, such as immunizations for children, prenatal care, and HIV and malaria intervention, for paltry sums – and I do mean, paltry.

In Malawi, public health spending in 2020 was as little as $34 USD per person per year for everything health-related. In 2019, per-capita health spending in either Nicaragua or Thailand might have been considered merely inadequate at $161 USD and $296 USD, respectively.[26] By contrast, Canada spent $6,666 USD, and the United States $13,590 USD on health care per person in the same year. Those numbers make it easier to understand why so many cervical cancer screening programs in lower-income countries remain unfunded, programs based only on name and good intention. I've helped a number of countries write their cervical cancer screening guidelines and I know those guidelines are still words on paper, waiting for the money to make them matter, even years after they've been written.

Volunteer "Firefighters": The Problem with NGOs

When countries can't afford cervical cancer screening, it's tempting to look to more affluent sources for solutions. One way lower-income governments can augment health care funding is to turn to external nongovernmental organizations (NGOs) or international development partners for assistance. These organizations and individuals can establish short-term, targeted programs for screening and treating women for cervical cancer, offering services to women who might otherwise have nothing. These pilot projects introduce the idea of routine screening, creating a degree of public awareness and demand. But in countries subject to scarcity, these approaches have their drawbacks.

Meaningfully addressing cervical cancer requires ongoing, universal, and sustainable screening programs. These goals are, frankly, incompatible with external aid, which is almost always short term in nature. During the period of a pilot project, for instance, women living in the project's targeted region will typically get screened for free or at minimal charge. But the governments in these countries are rarely able to absorb these short-term projects into their long-term health portfolios, or expend the resources needed to maintain these programs once the pilot is completed. And in the absence of a steady program for cervical cancer prevention – which only works when it's offered long-term – short-term solutions can damage citizens' confidence and trust.

In this sense, external aid against cervical cancer can create more problems than it solves: the use of development assistance to fill gaps in government health funding becomes a vicious cycle. Given the option of outside funding, governments with scarce resources can be tempted to consistently underfund health care programs in general, and cervical cancer screening programs in particular – despite their extraordinarily high rates of cervical cancer. When NGOs or development partners try to fill these gaps, the uncertainty surrounding funding creates a dynamic of distrust – and at worse, a cycle of dependency.

Dependency on unpredictable funding sources leads countries to chronically underplan and underfund health care budgets. It also contributes to a scarcity mentality among politicians and the public alike, where a lack of resources lowers expectations, which then fosters a lack of political will to make those resources a priority. As an obstetrician and medical researcher in Kenya, Dr. Mugo has developed her own sense of reticence toward NGO-funded programs. "If we make ourselves beggars and depend on partner funding, we do not get to prioritize our health agenda," she said. "The total impact of these [cervical cancer screening pilot] projects is not that large. In the wider ocean, it's a teaspoon."

In reference to the 2017 Kenyan study mentioned earlier in this chapter, a tiny fraction of local women sought cervical cancer screening despite Kenya's twenty-year commitment and plan for such services. The plan seemed to fall prey to inconsistent funding from the Kenyan government, which relied too heavily on limited external support. No short-term project with outside funding will correct this travesty. In Dr. Mugo's view – and mine – only a consistently funded program, which requires government's assurances of that commitment, can ensure that a country properly and universally addresses the spread of cervical cancer by screening.

When I was in Malawi in 2018, I had a chance to visit an NGO-funded cervical cancer screening project designed to screen 55,000 women. I was impressed with the industriousness and organizational skills of program developers and could see many women getting screened who would otherwise not have been able to do so. NGO facilitators were wisely working in a local public HIV care clinic, offering screening services to women coming to address other health needs: all positive benefits! I was, however, concerned that the NGO was not integrating into the public health system. When the project was over, would anything be sustained?

I worried it might not be, and here's why.

The NGO was using its own nurses for VIA screening, hiring its own doctors when surgery was needed for treatment, and even constructing its own operating theater separate from the local hospital. Apart from using a room in the local clinic to offer their services, program organizers were not integrating into the local health care system. The project even relied on imported cleaning materials and treatment equipment from outside the country. I was struck by the massive, expensive effort being put into developing a structure parallel to the existing cervical cancer screening system, and I suspected this service would likely vanish when the project was over. I could well understand Dr. Mugo's weariness for reliance on outside funding for a critical health need. This project was a boon for the 55,000 women being screened, but offered few assurances for improving local cervical cancer screening once the NGO left south-central Malawi.

This vicious cycle of dependency on outside funding repeats itself in many countries around the world. Not only is cervical cancer a hotly contested budget item within a country's internal budgeting processes, it also competes against other countries for international attention from external development agencies. All too often, the outside funder chooses where to spend its money, and along the line, the cause of cervical cancer misses out.

One U.S. study from 2020 found that in lower-income countries, 32 percent of health development assistance went toward "reproductive, maternal, newborn, and child health," while funding for noncommunicable diseases – including cancer and screening for cancer – received just 2 percent of funding, despite those diseases accounting for more than 62 percent of the global disease burden.[27] Maybe you are wondering, like I am, why reproductive health spending doesn't include cervical cancer care. The likelihood of lower-income countries accessing just 2 percent of an already negligible amount of donor funding gives new meaning to the word *scarce*.

Money, Money, Everywhere – and Still the "Fires" Burn

While having the financial resources on paper, higher-income countries face unique funding obstacles with regard to cervical cancer screening programs. As a result, even persons with cervixes living amid affluence struggle to stay on top of screening requirements. Per capita health spending in the United States is over $13,000 USD per person a year, but that amount is not offered to individuals equally. With no universal funding for health care, spending on health care varies greatly from state to state, and women on low incomes go without care in shocking ways, and with tragic results. As a doctor who's worked in a number of clinics servicing people who rely on state medical funding, I've seen firsthand the complex array of reasons women don't always get properly screened or treated for pre-cancer or cervical cancer – and poverty is the most disheartening of them all.

Angie was just such a patient at a clinic in Brownsville, Texas, where I worked after finishing my residency. While

I didn't see Angie myself, I did speak with her later about her experiences with cervical cancer. A petite woman with expressive brown eyes, Angie exuded warmth the first time I saw her. I immediately leaned into her story.

Angie first came to the Brownsville clinic when she was thirty-six years old. A single mother, she'd been working full-time in a nursing home for eleven dollars an hour while caring for her live-in mother and her own two children. Angie understood the importance of cervical cancer screening but had gotten behind on her Pap smears. With no health insurance from her job, she couldn't afford doctor visits.

Angie's situation is strikingly common in her state. As noted in Chapter 8, the 2018 study of the Rio Grande/Loredo, Texas border region, which includes Brownsville, found 70,000 women without health insurance.[28] This problem isn't limited to Texas. An estimated 7.9 million women in the United States lack health insurance – citizens who likely can't afford cervical cancer screening or follow-up unless they find a clinic offering subsidized services.[29]

In the United States, a Pap smear costs a minimum of $100 USD, including the clinic visit and processing. For patients without health insurance or access to a subsidized clinic, critical follow-up care, such as a colposcopy or biopsy, can cost upwards of $1,000 USD. In other words, for U.S. women trying to address pre-cancer early enough to avoid a devastating outcome, cost and access to specialist services can seriously get in the way of those goals.

Some clinics, like Angie's in Brownsville, offer sliding scales based on state government allotments, but when that funding runs out, patients must pay out of pocket or return the following year when the clinic's funds have been replenished. These funding delays allow undiagnosed cervical cancer to further advance before detection and discourage women from getting screened before it's too late. As a result, people like Angie are left vulnerable, subject to the low-cost or government-funded options particular to their state, which vary based on the governing majority and its preferences.

According to the Texas state legislature, Angie, despite her three dependents, made "too much money" to qualify for Medicaid. Her low income did allow her to receive a Pap smear at the Brownsville community clinic, which funded a limited number of free Pap smears every year. When Angie finally made it to the clinic one August afternoon, she was told it had used up its annual subsidy allotment. With the regular $100 USD fee well outside her budget, Angie made a mental note to come back in February the following year, a gift to herself for Valentine's Day.

Angie did get into the clinic that February for a routine exam and Pap smear, and, three days later, got what she calls "the phone call that changed my life." Like almost every woman I've spoken with who received a cervical cancer diagnosis, she could recall specific details even five years after the fact.

"I was sitting in the crowded break area for employees at the nursing home when the clinic called to tell me my Pap smear came back suspicious for cervical cancer." She paused as she spoke to me on screen, her eyes welling up. "I had to get up and turn off the TV playing in the break room to make sure I was hearing the words correctly. I remember asking the person on the phone if I was going to die, and thinking to myself, 'who would take care of my children and my mother?' For them, I was the only one."

Thankfully, Angie's screening test led to a biopsy, which confirmed her cancer was still in an early stage, and she received follow-up care. Ironically, it was only *after* she'd received a cancer diagnosis that she qualified for government-funded emergency insurance to cover her radiation treatment. Five years later, Angie is a cervical cancer survivor – and given her circumstances, she is one of the lucky ones.

The Kink in the Firehose: Politics Messing with Prevention

Of course, not all persons with cervixes are so "lucky." While Angie did ultimately get follow-up care and lifesaving treatment, limited access to affordable Pap screening placed her in a terrifying position. In 2010, in an effort to improve health care affordability for vulnerable citizens like Angie, the U.S. Congress passed the Affordable Care Act. Hoping to cast a wider safety net around women trying to prevent cervical cancer, the ACA mandated that all insurance companies pay for cervical cancer screening, including Medicaid, the federal and state program established in 1965 to help people on a lower income pay their health care expenses. Under the ACA, individual states could opt to expand their Medicaid coverage, increasing the number of residents in that state who qualified for funding, including coverage for cervical cancer screening. The key word here was *opt*.

Varying support for Medicaid expansion from state to state has meant that access to services like cervical cancer screening relies heavily on which state a woman lives in. I work in Washington, a state that chose to expand Medicaid, and thereby accepted the federal government income ceiling for individuals to qualify for Medicaid, which is one and a third times the federal poverty level. In 2022, for a family of four like Angie's living in Washington State, the family would qualify for Medicaid funding if the annual household income was less than $38,295 USD a year.[30] But Angie happened to live in Texas, a state whose government chose *not* to expand its Medicaid program.

The crucial question is whether states who've opted out of Medicaid expansion – Alabama, Florida, Georgia, Kansas, Mississippi, North Carolina, South Carolina, South Dakota, Tennessee, Texas, Wisconsin, and Wyoming – have both lower rates of cervical cancer screening and higher rates of cervical cancer. The not-so-surprising answers are "yes" and "yes." In a 2015 U.S. study, researchers found that uninsured women living in these states – who would have been insured under Medicaid expansion – fell behind on cervical cancer screening far more readily than those living in states supporting Medicaid expansion.[31] In fact, states that did not expand Medicaid reported some of the highest cervical cancer rates in the United States. These include Alabama, Florida, Texas, and

Mississippi – states with cervical cancer rates between 9 and 10 women per 100,000, and cervical cancer rates 70 percent greater than the U.S. national average and 1.5 times greater than those in Washington State.[32] In fact, consistent with years of reduced funding for cervical cancer screening, a 2022 U.S. national study showed that Stage 4 cervical cancer is actually increasing in the southern United States.[33]

The relationship between cervical cancer rates and lack of access to medical care implies that persons with cervixes in states without Medicaid expansion live (and die) at the mercy of state politics. U.S. politics – its divisiveness state to state – directly interferes with regular and proper screening to prevent cervical cancer. Nowhere has this link been more obvious than in the states who've recently chosen to defund their Planned Parenthood clinics, which have traditionally provided thousands of women with these vital, low-cost screening services.

The Fight over Abortion Lays Waste to Affordable Cancer Care

Remember Morgan from Chapter 9, whose life was rocked by an advanced cervical cancer diagnosis at just twenty-four? Morgan was diagnosed at a Planned Parenthood clinic, where she had gone for her routine cervical screening. According to the 2019 Planned Parenthood fact sheet, one in every five American women, like Morgan, has accessed a Planned Parenthood clinic for her health care. And, in Morgan's case, thank goodness she did. Planned Parenthood clinics provide nearly 500,000 Pap tests to 3 million patients every year. Between 2019 and 2020, those Pap tests gave early diagnoses to more than 75,000 women or identified them as at risk of developing cervical cancer. Many of Planned Parenthood's 3 million clients belong to marginalized groups; 15 percent of them are African American, and 24 percent, Latino.[34,35] When a political agenda defunds a clinic system providing lifesaving services to women – as Planned Parenthood defunding does in order to stop abortions – women are the ones who lose, their access to a lifesaving cancer test traded away for political gain.

U.S. state legislators have justified defunding clinics because they consider decreasing abortion access a priority. Yet, only 3 percent of Planned Parenthood's national budget goes toward terminating pregnancies, with none of the funds for abortion services coming directly from the public purse.[34] In responding first to antiabortion sentiment and overlooking the substantial role these clinics play in protecting women from disease, legislators have left their constituents with cervixes at deadly risk, and, as with declining Medicaid expansion, consigned health care needs to ever-changing political whims.

Scarcity Mindset: Why I Say No

When the WHO and its 194 member countries committed to eliminating cervical cancer worldwide, they also pledged to screen 70 percent of eligible persons with cervixes by 2030. The Union for International Cancer Control, PATH (a global public health organization), Gavi, the International Papillomavirus Society, and a multitude of other groups have joined this call to action.

But given the obstacles to widespread screening that we've covered, this goal can feel wildly aspirational. To reach it, we'll need better, cheaper screening tests, and enough adequately trained medical providers. We'll need more and better resources for follow-up treatment, without which a screening test is just a smoke alarm ringing while no one is home to hear it. We'll need more clinics, more supplies for clinics, and the ability to track and follow the numbers and outcomes of those attending the clinics. We'll need to address stigma and taboo, cultural context, racism, and gender bias with grassroots public education, as well as systemic change.

A daunting list indeed.

In order for countries to truly overcome these obstacles, their capacity to address cervical cancer will need to be examined, reexamined, and reimagined with energy, political will, and generous public health budgets. If cervical cancer screening acts like a kind of smoke alarm for detecting cancer, then we need to treat the elimination of this disease as a five-alarm blaze atop a very tall mountain.

So, my question is: Do we have enough energy? Do we have enough political will? Are our public health budgets generous enough? This chapter may have convinced you that the sad answer is no: that these challenges will always be ablaze atop that tall mountain looming ever present on the horizon. But for me, quitting – just as Ruth told me when I saw her that day in the Lilongwe clinic – is not an option. For Ruth, money was scarce. The number of trained health care providers was insufficient. Record-keeping was inadequate. Transportation was meager. She was anxious and afraid and overwhelmed. But she climbed that tall mountain because, as she said to me, she *had* to keep going, regardless of how she felt. Her family needed the money from her work, and her children needed their mother.

Our world needs Ruth and the hundreds of thousands of women like her who, every year, suffer through cervical cancer diagnoses, endure challenging treatments and their terrible side effects, and are often left with permanent and life-altering disfigurements and chronic health problems. Their contribution to families, communities, and nations is incalculable. Their loss is our loss. When we lose these women: their caregiving, their contributions, their wages, their energy and commitment, their *lives*, that is the real poverty – the true scarcity. I refuse to succumb to the mindset that there isn't enough, that there will never be enough. That "scarcity mindset" numbs me and slows me and lies to me. If I had asked my colleagues thirty years ago, "Do you think there will ever be a vaccine that can prevent cervical cancer?" we all would have said no – it's just not possible. If I had asked them, "Do you think one hundred and ninety-four countries around the world would commit to eliminating cervical cancer some day?" they would have said no, again.

We have enough to say, *Enough!* Let us keep asking for the energy, the political will, the funding to summit the mountain of cervical cancer elimination. And let the intrinsic worth of women be the bedrock for this effort. Let us ask ourselves every day: What is a woman worth? To me? To my community? To my country?

And let's take our cue from Ruth. Each day we can choose to continue mountain climbing, working to overcome these scarcities, working to establish sustainable, universal cervical screening programs, working to value women, working to save lives. Let us take one step at a time, encouraging each other as we climb, prodding each other when we want to give up.

Together, we can put out the fire at the top of that very tall mountain. The view from the top will be worth it.

12 "DYING INSIDE": OBSTACLES TO TREATMENT – AND THE CATASTROPHIC CONSEQUENCES

After discovering monumental obstacles to cervical cancer prevention, if you're reluctant to read about the travails of treatment, I sympathize. But it's only in learning about the hurdles women face in accessing treatment that we see the true toll of this disease. Indeed, it's in arriving at this desolate place that we stumble upon our deepest compassion.

As it turns out, the obstacles to treating cervical cancer are formidable, and the profound lack of treatment options worldwide lead to punishing outcomes for cervical cancer sufferers. It's worth repeating that right now, more than 340,000 women are dying or will die worldwide this year alone, dying for lack of treatment against a preventable disease. I cannot imagine a starker, more compelling argument for global HPV vaccination and deep investment in screening and treatment of precancer than the dearth of treatment services.

And yet each of these 340,000 women for whom vaccination, screening, or pre-cancer treatment came too late are crying out for lifesaving or even life-dignifying care.

The World Health Organization agrees. In 2019, the WHO's 194 member countries vowed to eliminate cervical cancer, and that strategy included 90 percent of women in need of treatment receiving "comprehensive management of invasive cervical cancer."[1] For me, these goals speak most to justice and human dignity. As noted in Chapter 8, 90 percent of all cervical cancer deaths occur in lower-income countries.[1] Not only do women living in lower-income countries receive the fewest cervical cancer protection options, but if they do get sick, their access to treatment – the kind offered in well-equipped, higher-income countries promising five-year survival for more than 80 percent of those diagnosed early – is infinitesimal.

In higher-income countries, treatment is tailored to address a cervical tumor's stage or spread. Typically, treatment involves radiation with possible chemotherapy, which requires specialized equipment and facilities and a radiation oncologist to plan the appropriate radiation dose and treatment. When cervical cancer is found early, with a less than four- to five-centimeter tumor confined to the cervix, surgery can eliminate it. But surgery, too, requires a specialized provider with advanced surgical training, and access to specialized resources like an operating room and hospital facilities. All of these treatment options can cure early-stage cancer and markedly improve and extend life even when the cancer isn't curable.

Unless you're one of the 90 percent.

Provision of these sophisticated types of equipment, surgical facilities, and trained medical providers is relatively rare among that "90 percent" in lower-income countries. Access to these resources is even more rare. Frankly, women in lower-income countries often struggle to receive medical care of any kind. For those living in rural or remote areas, going to a doctor or a clinic outside of pregnancy is often seen as unnecessary. Instead, cervical cancer acts like a ticking time bomb, with women seeking care only after they've developed visible symptoms: persistent vaginal bleeding; ongoing, foul-smelling vaginal discharge; severe back pain; or leg swelling. These signs usually suggest Stage 3 or 4 cancer, at which point, persons with cervixes in these parts of the world are lucky to have one of two options: a diminished form of treatment to prolong their lives for a few months or more, or, if they can afford it, private treatment in another country at a very steep price.

The overwhelming reality, then, is that cervical cancer patients in lower-income countries will die excruciatingly painful deaths, sometimes isolated from family or friends because of stigma or the noxious smell of a cervix filled with dying tissue. In their final days, they are often bereft of palliative care. Once again, scarcity equals suffering.

As a young medical student, I received a firsthand introduction to the catastrophic consequences of meager resources for treating cervical cancer in lower-income countries. It was an experience that haunts me to this day.

Meeting Mama

At twenty-five, I traveled to a clinic and affiliated hospital outside Monrovia, Liberia, for my last rotation in my final year of medical school: a four-month, clinical learning rotation in family medicine. Having just flown across the Atlantic for the first time, and still awash in the fog of jet lag, I was on my second day working in a clinic when I encountered a patient whose gentle face I still recall. At that time, much of my surroundings were new to me: women walking around in flip-flops and colorful skirts toting babies bound to their backs by rectangular pieces of brightly patterned cloth; the smells of fried bread and roasting goat hanging from the racks of street vendors near the clinic; the foreign cadence and tones of languages I didn't know. It was exhilarating and overwhelming.

But my overriding desire to care for patients had brought me halfway across the world to Africa, and that motivation grounded me. Not quite done with medical school, I was there to learn and share whatever skills and knowledge I could offer. My goal was to join with a team of medical providers permanently based in Liberia to offer the best possible care. This was a time of rapid, almost dizzying, growth for me as I tried to take it all in. Between patient visits at the clinic, I would peer out into the waiting room, wondering if we were making a dent in the long line of patients. One afternoon, I noticed a woman and a man I assumed to be her grown son sitting beside each other.

No one sat beside them, even though the other benches were squeezed full, with many patients standing. I noted the unusual sight and kept working.

About an hour later, my supervising physician, Dr. Steve Befus, asked me to accompany him tending to a patient. I followed him eagerly down the hall toward a patient examining room. Halfway there, I stopped in my tracks, almost knocked off balance by a smell – a putrid, rotten odor. Dr. Befus continued walking, seemingly oblivious. I quickly regained my composure and hurried to catch up. As we reached the examination room, the smell became overpowering. I walked in and recognized the woman and her grown son who'd been sitting alone in the waiting room. I understood. The smell had allowed them a bench to themselves.

The woman was sitting fully clothed on a bare exam table, her hands folded on her lap. Her high cheekbones stood out against her pale, gaunt face and her shoulder bones poked through her thin, white T-shirt, unevenly tucked into the tie-dyed cloth she'd wrapped around her slight waist as a skirt. Our eyes met. I smiled at her, and right away she looked down. *Had I been too direct? As a twenty-five-year-old medical student, was I not showing enough respect to this mature woman?* This was only my second day in Liberia. I worried my eye contact and direct smile had been a cultural faux pas.

Her son, who looked to be in his mid-twenties, spoke up from the folding chair at the end of the exam table. "She is embarrassed because of her smell," he explained. His dark eyes were pools of sadness. He looked first at Dr. Befus, and then at me. "She did not want to come, but we are all worried about her. We want to know what is wrong."

I watched Dr. Befus address this dignified, gray-haired woman with deep compassion. "Mama," he said, using an endearment I would later learn Liberians and long-standing guests in the country use to address elderly women, "we are here to try to help. Would you let us look to try to understand what is happening with your body?"

"Mama" looked away, focused on some distant spot. We waited, all of us enveloped by that rotten odor, grabbing at small sips of air.

Her son spoke, almost begging: "Mama, please let them try."

After a long pause, Mama said to us, "The smell is too strong," and, almost as an afterthought, "I am dying inside."

Dr. Befus gently touched Mama's shoulder. "We can check to see if we can help," he told her. Mama turned to look at her son, who was staring at her with pleading eyes, and nodded her assent.

Dr. Befus and I covered her with a sheet and helped her lie back on the table. After checking above her collar bones, and in the inguinal (groin) area of her lower abdomen to see if her lymph nodes were enlarged, Dr. Befus gently raised her skirt, folding her knees open. The smell became overpowering. I suppressed a wave of nausea and Mama bent her thin arm over her head, hiding her face in the crook of her elbow. Her son looked at the floor, clearly trying to protect his mother's privacy. The odor in the air mingled with their shared shame.

Dr. Befus placed a gloved finger inside her vagina. After about fifteen seconds, he removed his finger and stood back. We covered Mama's body again with the sheet, and Dr. Befus looked over at me, his face somber. I gave Mama a cloth she could use to clean herself, and he and I stepped out in the hall to allow her to get dressed.

"She has cervical cancer," Dr. Befus said. "The cancer has spread down the back of her vagina and up under her bladder." He paused, looking away for a moment, and, although I did not yet know him well, I thought I saw tears welling up in his eyes. After a deep breath, Dr. Befus seemed to come back, his face composed and his speech again calm and professional.

"I saw another patient last week with a similar odor. She also had cervical cancer," he said. "We don't have any treatment we can offer her."

"Can't we help her at all?" I said, my thoughts slamming up against this newfound reality of working in Liberia, far away from fully equipped American medical centers where I had spent all of my previous training.

"We can try to make her more comfortable. We will give her some pain medicine and try some antibiotics to see if we can help lessen the vaginal odor. Her odor is a sign of her tissue dying from cancer."

He paused and looked at me, offering one last thought before we went back into the room.

"You will never forget this patient."

Dr. Befus was right. I have never forgotten her.

I have also never forgotten what it was like to go back into that treatment room and watch Mama and her son receive the news that she had advanced cancer, and that Liberia could offer her no treatment. Her previously stoic son began to cry and Mama, regaining her regal composure, asked her son to take her home to be with her family. Then she looked Dr. Befus directly in the eye. "I knew it was my time to die," she told him. "I did not want to waste our family money for me to come."

"You will never forget this patient."
Dr. Befus was right. I have never forgotten her.
I have also never forgotten what it was like to go back into that treatment room and watch Mama and her son receive the news that she had advanced cancer, and that Liberia could offer her no treatment.

One for One Thousand: The Steep Climb for a Cure

I met Mama in 1987. I wish I could say that there are no longer places like Liberia was then, where a woman would not know she had cervical cancer until she felt she was "dying inside." But there remain too many *Mamas* today: women with advanced cervical cancer and no options at all for treatment, including palliative care. What gets in the way of their basic human right to care and deserved dignity is, once again, about scarcity – the absence of *enough* skilled providers, *enough* specialized equipment, *enough* cultural, social, and financial support.

In lower-income countries, the lack of oncologists – doctors with expertise in cancer care treatment – is a widespread, well-documented problem. The relative scarcity of medical providers with expertise in oncology was the subject of a 2018 India–U.S. research report that looked at ninety-three countries around the globe, including high-, middle-, and low-income countries.[2] The researchers noted an "extreme shortage" – defined as a single oncologist needing to see more than a thousand new cancer patients per year – in twenty-five countries in Africa and one country (Sri Lanka) in Asia. Eight countries had no oncologists at all.[3] By contrast, none of the countries of Europe or North or South America faced an "extreme shortage" of clinical oncologists.

It's important to note that this survey looked at the availability of oncologists in general and didn't account for the greater scarcity of gynecologic oncologists, doctors trained to do essential treatments like radical hysterectomies and lymph node dissections. But it certainly exposed the lack of skilled cancer care providers in countries needing them most (Figure 12.1).

My Malawian colleague Dr. Lameck Chinula may have received the training necessary to perform radical hysterectomies, but he is the only physician in northern Malawi trained to do so – and one of just five doctors qualified to surgically treat cervical cancer in this country of over 19 million. When I spoke with Dr. Chinula in May 2022, his patients faced a four-month wait to get on his surgery schedule. For those whose tumors are too big for surgery, Dr. Chinula told me, "I am desperately working with my clinical oncologist colleagues to be able to give women chemotherapy. We are yet to have any radiation treatment available in Malawi."

Dr. Chinula's challenges are far from extraordinary. While working in Namibia, I discovered that the country of South Africa offered the only option for Namibian women who needed surgery for cervical cancer. This treatment option would require patients to cover the costs of medical attention, travel,

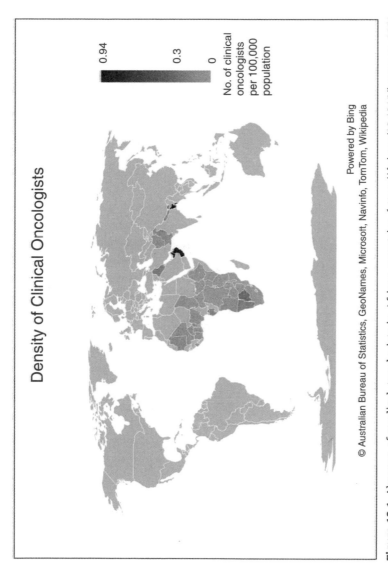

Density of Clinical Oncologists

0.94

0.3

0

No. of clinical
oncologists
per 100,000
population

Powered by Bing

© Australian Bureau of Statistics, GeoNames, Microsoft, Navinfo, TomTom, Wikipedia

Figure 12.1 Absence of medical oncologists in African countries. https://doi.org/10.1016/j.esmoop.2021
.100292 1

and leaving behind their families – an impossible feat for local women struggling to make ends meet.

Though cervical cancer sufferers in higher-income countries face far less dire circumstances, gynecologic oncologists can be in short supply there as well. These specialists, who are critical to managing a patient's treatment, require an additional four years of training beyond that of an obstetrician gynecologist. And yet, the aforementioned global India–U.S. study estimated by 2025 a U.S. shortage of 2,300 medical oncologists.[2] The Society of Gynecologic Oncology of Canada estimates that its current number of working members is about half the number needed to support the next decade's anticipated population growth.[3]

Mountains beyond Mountains: Scarcity of Equipment and Supplies

Practicing medical providers worldwide already face challenges beyond an excess of patients and too few hours in the day. Cervical cancer treatment requires use of a computerized tomography (CT) scan to assess disease spread, radiotherapy equipment for treating and curing disease, operating rooms, and blood supplies for surgery.* Summiting the mountain of treatment challenges can lead to falls and false starts at any stage of this journey.

In many countries, accessing a CT scan requires an arduous, expensive journey to an urban center where one might be available but not necessarily working. My Zambian colleague

---

* A CT scan creates a more detailed picture than a regular X-ray by using computer processing to combine a series of X-ray images of the inside of the body taken from various angles. CT scans are often used to detect the spread of cervical cancer and the presence of disease in lymph nodes. Magnetic resonance imaging (MRI) is a type of diagnostic test that can create detailed images of nearly every structure and organ inside the body. Rather than relying on radiation, an MRI uses magnets and radio waves to produce images on a computer. Images produced by an MRI scan can show organs, bones, muscles, and blood vessels.
"CT Scan vs. MRI: What's the Difference? And How Do Doctors Choose Which Imaging Method to Use?" Memorial Sloan Kettering Cancer Center, 2022, accessed March 20, 2023. www.mskcc.org/news/ct-vs-mri-what-s-difference-and-how-do-doctors-choose-which-imaging-method-use.

Dr. Leeya Pinder had many cervical cancer patients arrive in Lusaka to find the CT scanner broken and awaiting repair. The losses of work and wages, the expenses of the journey, and the dashed hopes became their own deterrents to patient care. Some women, Dr. Pinder told me, "just didn't come back."

Patients who've overcome logistics around seeking and receiving care, who've had their disease spread mapped, and who've acquired a skilled treatment provider go on to face, as the Haitian proverb goes, "more mountains beyond mountains." You may remember Elvia and Kim from Chapter 8, friends whose cervical cancer outcomes were directly dependent on where they lived. In the United States, Kim had immediate access to care and was cured. In Haiti, a country with no radiation machines, Elvia only received a diagnosis. She died a few months later. Elvia's story plays out over and over around the world every year.

Dr. Chinula points to a similar situation in Malawi: no radiation machines anywhere for treating people with cervical cancer. Patients are instead advised to travel to India for radiotherapy. For citizens of Malawi – a country ranked 180th out of 190 for its Gross Domestic Product – a trip to India is like suggesting a trip to the moon.

Some lower-income countries have radiation equipment, but not enough radiation oncologists to operate it. In 2017, when I was in Namibia working on the country's cervical cancer guidelines, the country's sole radiation oncologist grappled continually with equipment shortages. The number of advanced cervical cancer patients needing emergent radiation for serious vaginal bleeding was so great, she told me, she could only control their bleeding with palliative radiation. She couldn't trade the pressing needs of urgent care patients to try to cure women with early cervical cancer, although she was glad to make dying women more comfortable. "But I really wish I was getting to treat them much earlier," she told me, "when I could potentially save their lives."

A 2017 report by the International Atomic Energy Agency confirms the dearth of radiotherapy for individuals living in lower-income countries.[4] In higher-income countries, one radiotherapy machine is available for every 120,000 people. But in lower-income countries, a single radiotherapy machine can be expected to serve about 5 million people. Think about that: 5 *million*. This same report found that only twenty-one of forty-eight sub-Saharan African radiotherapy facilities offer any radiotherapy – radiotherapy equipment requires maintenance, which requires parts and technicians these clinics don't have or can't afford.

More scarcity. More suffering.

In August 2020, I spoke about these radiotherapy treatment challenges with Dr. Lynette Denny, a gynecologic oncologist who started the South African oncology program in Cape Town. In Dr. Denny's experience, "typically even if there might be nine facilities, only two of them will be working." When radiotherapy machines break down, she explained, it can be difficult to find replacement parts or skilled expertise to repair them. In November 2022, I learned that Uganda's sole radiation machine – in the country's only cancer treatment center in Kampala – had remained broken for two years. The implication was that no women in Uganda had access to local radiation treatment until recently, when the machine was finally repaired and brought back into operation. Even if a lower-income region has a radiation machine, there is no guarantee radiation treatment is available – unless that machine comes with a trained provider and is operating well enough to be of use.

The Forbidding Peak of Treatment

After the "mountains beyond mountains" comes the most unsettling blight on the horizon: treatment for cervical cancer.

If a person with a cervix has climbed all of these mountains – screening, diagnosis, CT mapping, and oncological access – the radiation treatment regimen presents an uphill battle few are prepared to face. Radiation requires daily therapy, typically for five days a week and a total of twenty-five to thirty-five

treatments. The expense of such a regimen is often impractic-
able and unaffordable for many patients. What's more, unless
a woman lives where the radiation is being offered, she'll have
to pay for nearby lodging to receive it and be away from family
for a prolonged period. For women who serve as their family's
central caregivers, income earners, or both, such treatment
requirements can be socially, emotionally, and financially
impossible to meet.

Dr. Denny sees the difficulty local women experience in
completing their cervical cancer therapies and the consequent
implications for their suffering and survival. Once she'd finished her oncology training: "we were seeing ten women
a week with advanced cervical cancer and the survival rate of
our patients with cervical cancer was only thirty percent." Both
Dr. Denny and I knew that in higher-income countries, by
contrast, the cervical cancer survival rate was closer to
70 percent.

When Dr. Denny began investigating the clinic's low survival
rates, she found that only 45 percent of patients were completing radiation treatments. "Patients just could not stay away
from their homes that long," she said. "Sixty percent of them
are the sole breadwinners of their families. We found if they
ever went back home during their treatment for a visit, they
were very unlikely to return." Dr. Denny's experiences suggest
that a chance at survival means little without time or money to
complete treatment.

Government-funded health plans or private insurers often
fund treatment expenses in higher-income countries. In
Canada, Australia, and the United Kingdom, where citizens
enjoy universal health care, cancer treatment costs are typically
covered. In the United States, which lacks a publicly funded
medical system, a cervical cancer diagnosis grants state-
funded emergency medical insurance coverage for treatment,
particularly for those lacking personal or employer-funded
insurance. Although government emergency insurance typically pays for most cervical cancer treatments, it's not accepted
at all hospitals. It also represents a potentially deadly barrier to

care. Once cervical cancer patients receive treatment and achieve remission, they are no longer eligible, creating a potential lapse in care for women least likely to afford further medical tests, visits, and scans, and just when they most need close follow-up to prevent or manage recurrences. As a woman nears the summit of eliminating her cervical cancer, she sees her prognosis fall into a crevasse created by a country that – first and foremost – values self-sufficiency.

It's worth noting that even those lucky enough to have private insurance don't always receive coverage for gynecologic oncologists. A 2018 U.S. medical report found that 27 to 44 percent of women lacked access to a gynecologic oncologist as part of their insurance provider's approved physician network.[5] While gynecologic oncologists are best suited to treat cervical cancer, patients unable to pay "out-of-network" premiums may find themselves with substandard care and a lower likelihood of survival.

Cancer found early can sometimes be addressed via surgery. And yet, all of the obstacles we've discussed can stand in the way of surgical treatment as well: a lack of skilled providers, inadequate facilities and equipment, even limited blood supply. Because women can lose vaginal blood prior to surgery, and because radical hysterectomies usually involve blood loss, these surgeries require donated blood for transfusions. Many hospitals in lower-income countries lack the ability to collect and store blood easily, requiring family members to donate as necessary. Even in countries where surgeons and operating rooms are available, lifesaving radical hysterectomies can hinge on a scarcity as simple as insufficient blood.

Chemotherapy is one of the few treatment options more readily available in lower-income countries, but it's neither easier nor even particularly successful compared with surgery or radiation. Patients (such as Ruth in Chapter 11, who underwent chemotherapy for a cancer she didn't have) typically must find their own doctors experienced in administering chemotherapy, leading them toward the previously discussed challenges: a dearth of skilled providers, geographic barriers to providers, and, as ever, the inability to pay for it all. Patients are often responsible for procuring the necessary supplies: needles and tubing for intravenous delivery and the associated anti-cancer drugs. Rarely do people in lower-income countries have access to the newer, cancer-fighting chemotherapy agents that higher-income countries enjoy, such as the potent and versatile Bevacizumab. Instead, they must rely on older and far less effective chemotherapy drugs, still in no way as efficacious as radiation therapy.

Traveling for Treatment: Another Looming Challenge

Geographic access to any type of cervical cancer treatment is a challenge in lower- and higher-income countries alike. If a country does have the right providers and equipment, they are often located in urban areas. For persons with cervixes who live in rural or remote areas, poor roads, deserts, mountains, swollen rivers during rainy seasons, long, impassable distances, or unreliable or simply unavailable transportation all present definitive obstacles. These factors can delay or even discourage women from initial treatment and follow-up, and ultimately undermine their survival.

Studies show that gynecological cancer patients who rely on gynecologic oncologists rather than general surgeons or gyne-cologists typically experience timelier, better treatment and superior survival rates.[6] But medical training programs for gynecologic oncologists are usually located in urban centers. Since many health care providers end up settling and working where they train, fully trained gynecologic oncologists tend to be centered in urban areas, making already scarce specialists even less accessible to rural cancer patients. In the United States, 72 percent of gynecologic oncologists practice in urban settings, and 43 percent at university hospitals. Only 13 percent of gynecologic oncologists practice in areas with populations below 50,000.

Geographic inequities are not unique to the United States. Western Australia and the Australian state of Tasmania, both of which encompass significant land masses, have just one gynecological oncology center.[7] Neither the Northern Australia Territory nor the Australian Capital Territory has a gynecological treatment unit to treat women with cervical cancer. This scarcity of specialists leaves large numbers of Australian cervical cancer patients without the critical expertise for treatment unless they have the time, money, and wherewithal to travel long distances to find it.

Texas Is Kind of Big, Ya Know

In the spring of 1990, while in residency training at the University of Texas MD Anderson Cancer Center in Houston, I met a patient named Linda. We hit it off immediately – perhaps because we shared the same first name!

Linda was fifty-three, nearly twice my age at the time, and had been at MD Anderson three years earlier for radiation treatment of Stage 2A cervical cancer. She was back again because her hometown clinic in El Paso had just diagnosed her with a recurrence. El Paso lies 750 miles west of Houston.

As I opened the door to the exam room, my usual greeting of "Hello, I'm Doctor Eckert!" went unacknowledged. My 9:00 a.m. patient was sound asleep, curled up on the exam table and snoring under two white sheets she must have retrieved from the storage cabinet in the corner of the room before converting them into a pillow. She was not alone: a younger woman sat slumped in a chair, her head leaning against the wall and mouth wide open, also sound asleep. I hated to wake them; they obviously needed the rest.

I finally placed my hand gently on Linda's shoulder to let her know I was there, and she startled, pushing herself up to sitting. "Oh my . . . so embarrassing . . . I'm so sorry," she said, her loud voice waking her companion. "I must've really needed a nap."

I offered each of them a glass of water and we introduced ourselves. I learned that the woman in the chair was Linda's neighbor, Rose, who had driven Linda through the night to get to this appointment. "I had to finish my work shift," Rose said. "We didn't have time to stop and get some shut-eye." She smiled. "I guess I was so tired that even this stiff chair couldn't keep me awake."

Linda didn't drive. The eleven-hour trip to Houston represented a severe hardship, one she endured because MD Anderson, the largest cancer hospital in the United States, offered cancer care to all Texas residents regardless of insurance status. Her job as a home health care provider didn't come with private medical insurance. This was Linda's only treatment option.

During her previous radiation treatment, MD Anderson had provided Linda an apartment to stay in during her multiple daily treatment sessions. But she hadn't been back to our clinic for follow-up visits in more than two years. "I came to my appointments in the first year, but after that, I just couldn't get here." When I asked why, she simply shrugged and said, "Texas is kind of big, ya know." She and Rose looked at each other and smiled, and I could see their mutual affection. It seemed clear to me that if not for the help of this caring neighbor, Linda wouldn't have made this visit at all. "I couldn't afford the bus ticket," she said, "so Rose, bless her heart, offered to drive me." She looked at Rose, and I thought I saw some tears in Linda's eyes as she said, "Now *that* is a neighbor for you."

At twenty-seven, and in the very beginning of my career, I was shocked to hear of the great distance Linda had to travel to receive cancer treatment. But as I continued in my rotation at MD Anderson, I would meet many such patients as Linda. And while some, like Linda, could get housing in Houston to attend their initial treatments, critical follow-up appointments presented another level of difficulty. When recurrences are found earlier, women live longer.[8] A 2016 University of Alabama study found that cervical cancer patients living more than 100 miles from a major referral hospital experienced much lower longevity (an average span of five-and-a-half years) than those living less than 100 miles away (an average span of eight years, three months). A 2015 study of 150 women with gynecologic cancers receiving care at Baltimore's University of Maryland found that those needing to travel more than 50 miles were less likely to complete their care.[9]

I work at the University of Washington in Seattle, which, in addition to serving Washington residents, serves as the referral medical center for Alaska, whose land mass represents 30 percent of the entire United States, and whose interior is often entirely without roads. When women in remote areas of Alaska need treatment for cervical cancer, they must travel by plane to major clinics in Anchorage or Seattle. It's not hard to imagine the cost and time for these trips deterring women from seeking care.

For women with few financial resources, regardless of citizenship, the hardships of traveling for treatment – time off work, the cost and availability of transportation and lodging, childcare – further complicate an ever-present challenge.

Limited access to cancer specialists and clinics amplifies the vulnerability for women living in rural or remote areas. These patients are statistically less likely to adhere to typical cervical cancer prevention routines for the same reasons they might not access treatment. They're less likely to receive a timely diagnosis or access treatment, translating to more suffering, and more death.

Private Parts, Property, and Prejudice: When Stigma and Bias Preempt Care

If the stigma around investigating a "private" body part like a cervix gets in the way of cancer screening, that same stigma turns treatment into impassable terrain. As my Kenyan colleague Dr. Mugo said, "Women do not discuss their private parts." Taboo around female anatomy in a country like Kenya can result in a woman being cast out of her tight-knit community, unable to work, even losing her home or place to stay. This taboo assumes a deadly form in communities where a husband considers a woman's body his domain, and only he is allowed to see it. If a cervical exam is considered a violation, the quest for treatment stops before it has begun. Furthermore, if a woman's body is seen as property, then a dramatic bodily threat or disfigurement reduces its "value" or "utility." From this vantage, a cervical cancer diagnosis magnifies the trauma for its sufferers and survivors. "Lack of social support, most importantly from spouses," states the WHO in its strategy to eliminate cervical cancer, "has the greatest adverse impact on quality of life of women cancer survivors in sub-Saharan Africa."

Given the stigma toward female reproductive cancers, women might forgo treatment in order to delay inevitable social losses. For women like Mama, the odor of advanced cervical cancer is like a scarlet "C" that a woman cannot take off. What's more, during an already terrible time, the unmistakable smell of necrotic tissue can leave a woman with cervical cancer isolated from the people she needs most, less likely to overcome shame and seek treatment, and bereft of the emotional support she'll need to endure it.

Dr. Mugo is well acquainted with the stigma of cervical cancer. When I spoke with her in late 2020, she recalled an advanced cervical cancer patient from thirty years earlier, a memory she says will never leave her, much the way Mama has never left me. "The woman was thirty-five or thirty-six at the time, had always been healthy, with a three-month-old baby, and a few other children," Dr. Mugo said. One of her colleagues asked Dr. Mugo if she could fit this patient into her clinic schedule that day. "She was three months postpartum, and still having bleeding, so I told my colleague to have the patient come."

"When this woman arrived, I did an examination," Dr. Mugo recalled. "And I still, to this day, can see that examination. The tumor had eaten up all of her cervix and was coming down her vagina. She had advanced cancer."

"But," Dr. Mugo continued, "what was really shocking was what happened to her socially. The patient went home to her husband, who asked her what he was supposed to do with a wife

who could not be with him. What was he supposed to do with
a woman who was not useful in the bedroom?

"He kicked her out and sent her to a room back behind the
house, alone, and he took in another woman. I think she died
quickly, only lasting about three months," Dr. Mugo said. "I asked
another friend of mine about her children recently as I was thinking about her story. Her children never finished school."

The fear and misunderstanding around cervical cancer can
morph into deep-rooted judgments about the disease and its
sufferers. And the persistence of stigma can create biases
against the benefits of preventing or treating it, leading
women to delay or avoid consulting with medical providers.
But these destructive biases can go both ways. Although
a pelvic exam is essential to cervical cancer diagnosis and treatment, a shocking number of providers do not provide them, and
this, in part, can be attributed to "provider bias."

We've talked twice now about Teolita, a Black American
woman who went to the emergency room with abnormal bleeding two times in six months, but never received a pelvic examination until she saw a gynecologist. I wondered if an
unconscious or conscious bias about Teolita's skin color may
have led to assumptions that her bleeding was caused by an
infection or fibroids of the uterus. I wondered if – based on
proven harms associated with medical biases – these assumptions might have reduced the sense of urgency to examine
Teolita. But because Teolita came to the ER twice complaining
of vaginal bleeding, she was twice robbed of the opportunity to
detect her cancer earlier through a pelvic examination.

In South Africa, Dr. Denny observed that a woman can typically go to a health care provider an average of eight times
complaining of vaginal odor, bleeding, or pain before that provider offers an examination. She may receive antibiotics for
a presumed vaginal infection or some other type of treatment,
but without a pelvic examination, the true cause of her symptoms remains undiagnosed. A study of women with cervical
cancer in South Africa found urban women waited a year, on
average, between their first contact with a health provider and

a pelvic examination revealing cervical cancer; the wait was over two years for those living in rural areas.[10,11] Again, conscious or unconscious provider bias may lead to the presumption of vaginal discharge coming from an infection and the omission of that all-important pelvic examination signaling cervical cancer – delays that can make the difference between a curable cancer and a deadly, advanced one.

Patient shame can make it challenging to willingly surrender to a pelvic examination. Susie, my Harborview patient in Chapter 1 who presented with advanced cervical cancer, had put off her examination, hoping her vaginal odor would improve. Mama, in Chapter 11, endured shame and scorn from the vaginal odor caused by her cancer. These powerful feelings and attitudes – deterrents to seeking care – can be magnified by a history of socially sanctioned, internalized racism. Dr. Denny has had patients say, "I cannot tell a White man I have a smelly discharge," and "I cannot let a White man touch me." Dr. Denny considers these suspicions one of the long-lasting blights of apartheid.

Racial differences show up not just in the diagnosis of cervical cancer, but also in how and when and how much treatment a woman is offered. In the Tuskegee study mentioned in the last chapter, the authors noted that race played a part in the treatment options patients received after diagnosis.[12] These differences were most marked for Black women in rural areas as compared with White, urban women and they led to stark consequences: researchers partially attributed lower survival rates among Black women to less aggressive cancer treatments; they were more likely to receive radiation treatment and less likely to be offered surgery. The study found inequitable treatment options may reflect a lack of consistent, reliable health insurance but also systemic racial bias. A 2014 study conducted in Maryland uncovered the same treatment disparities: Black women were not receiving surgical treatment for cervical cancer as often as were White women.[13] In fact, while these studies did not report the reasons for these treatment differences, both the Alabama and Maryland studies found that even at the same stage of disease, White women were more likely to receive surgery.

The type of cervical cancer treatment offered to White versus non-White women is not the only notable distinction. Researchers have found evidence of racial differences correlating to delayed starting times between diagnosis and treatment. A 2022 University of California at San Diego study noted that Hispanic women were over two-and-a-half times more likely than White women to experience delays greater than seventy-five days between a cervical cancer diagnosis and the start of treatment.[14] When studies such as these spotlight inequities in cervical cancer treatment for those with non-White skin, then we need to consciously undo these differences and move toward equity-conscious cervical cancer care.

Cancer Risks Rise for Patients Denied Pelvic Exams

Delayed access to pelvic examinations doesn't just deny patients' urgent care. It also dangerously interrupts systemic efforts to eliminate the spread of disease. Pelvic exams provide an important tracking mechanism for cervical cancer rates. If a woman dies of cervical cancer before receiving a pelvic exam, a definitive diagnosis cannot be noted, skewing the picture of a country's cervical cancer suffering. No pelvic exam means no data. And when lack of data obscures the disease toll, public and government support for vaccination, screening, and treatment funding can falter. Without accurate counts of cervical cancer diagnoses and deaths, governments make spending decisions without urgency, catastrophically allowing the disease to persist and grow. Without data, national health ministries struggle to advocate for the very pelvic exams that lead to treatment perpetuating a vicious cycle.

When stigma and bias delay pelvic exams, they give cancer time to grow and put a woman at great risk for poorer outcomes. When stigma and bias prevent pelvic exams altogether, they cause – there's no gentle way to say this – death.

Alone and in Agony: The Absence of Palliative Care

We would like all girls in every country to receive the HPV vaccine. We all support widespread screening and treatment of pre-cancers for persons with cervixes so that fewer must experience cervical cancer treatment at all. Governments around the world would like to avoid the expense of more clinics, more specialty doctors, and more specialized equipment to treat this dreaded disease. Every WHO member country that committed to the elimination of cervical cancer understands the logic of these calculations.

But until women stop getting cervical cancer, we need treatment options, here and now. For the 600,000 women each year for whom vaccination, screening, or pre-cancer treatment has come too late, treatment is a human right and a deserved dignity. Persons with cervixes deserve timely pelvic examinations; access to gynecologic oncologists and skilled surgeons; specialized, well-maintained equipment; and, most of all, communities and governments that support these fundamental things with money and time and energy.

When women go without humane health care, they experience something akin to family or community shunning. When countries allow scarcity to deny them, they are further victimized by social repudiation – a communal disregard for pain and suffering.

As I write, I think once again of the mountain we all face in trying to eliminate cervical cancer, and I wonder: do we have enough to give women what they deserve?

Humanity and Compassion: The Quest to Dig Deep

Can we overcome scarcity? We must. And we can start on this fraught path by tackling the opportunity for universal "death with dignity." I'm talking about palliative care. Without it, the last weeks and months of a cervical cancer patient's life are always ones of relentless pain and suffering, sometimes exacerbated by isolation from her community and even her own family – always with the knowledge that society deems her unworthy, even of alleviating her pain, of giving her comfort in her final days. It seems trite to say that it doesn't have to be this way.

Palliative treatment for pain or bleeding allows women to die more peacefully. The establishment, strengthening, and integration of palliative care into cervical cancer treatment tells women and society that they are worth – at the very least – a death with dignity. That in the face of scarcity, comfort and caring always find a way. Given proper pain management, women are more likely to die among their loved ones, rather than alone in a room at the back of a house. It doesn't seem too much to ask for a way to offer the *Mamas* of the world a compassionate détente with the thief of cervical cancer.

That the suffering and death of so many *Mamas* goes unaddressed burns a fire inside me that propels me to write this book. My twenty-five-year-old medical student's heart wants cervical cancer treatment for all. And why not? The current state of cervical cancer treatment in lower-income countries should be unacceptable to anyone who believes in human dignity and worth. My now well-seasoned medical provider's heart sees the challenges but will not give up my belief in the value of all people. At bare minimum, I want palliative care for the women we cannot save, and I want their suffering to spur us on to the day when equitable, accessible treatment for cervical cancer, regardless of a country's income level or political affiliations, is a reality.

I remember saying plaintively to Dr. Befus so many years ago outside Mama's exam room, "Can't we help her at all?!"

Surely, we have enough for that.

13 WHAT MONEY CANNOT BUY

In a part of the world that values women for their ability to attract husbands and bear children, Barbara, a forty-one-year-old resident of Zimbabwe, is a divorced single woman – as well as an author, blogger, and trained counselor (Figure 13.1). She is also a survivor. Barbara, who endured fourteen surgeries to address her cervical cancer, has suffered unimaginably under a patriarchal system – but she hasn't allowed those terms to define her.

Yet her experiences remain a humbling reminder of the indignities women endure simply to stay alive.

With her head covered in a brown-toned, multihued scarf, warm eyes and ready smile apparent, Barbara shared her cervical cancer story with me via videoconference one September evening from her home in the southern region of Africa. She was just twenty-nine, she told me, married and living in Namibia, when posters on the walls of a hospital where she volunteered for women with breast cancer prompted her to go for a Pap smear. A few years earlier, her results had been normal. "I definitely was not expecting it when my Pap smear came back showing cervical cancer."

"After that," she said. "Everything moved so fast." Barbara was married to a physician. "He arranged everything, and I went quickly to a gynecologist. Because I had not had any children, my husband and the gynecologist decided it was best to just take a piece of my cervix." Her doctor's strategy was unorthodox – typically used only for microscopic-sized cancers – to place maximum emphasis on protecting Barbara's reproductive organs. "I was trying to get pregnant," Barbara recalled. "But it did not happen."

The focus on maintaining Barbara's fertility seemed to take precedence over fighting her cancer. Her gynecologist refused to give her chemotherapy or radiation. "Instead, I kept having surgery after surgery to remove the cancer whenever it came back." Trying to make sense of this unusual treatment plan, I asked Barbara to shed more light on her surgical ordeal. After all, cancer this persistent over so many years typically spreads and becomes lethal. "It turned out that I had endometriosis, as well as cervical cancer. They removed some of the endometriosis and some of the cancer," she said. "I kept having abnormal scans and surgery. Whenever they saw something abnormal on the scan, I would have another surgery."

Out of Barbara's fourteen surgeries, four of them were laparotomies, and ten, laparoscopies, all requiring general anesthesia and thereby putting her at risk. Each anesthesia amplified her chances of surgical complications – some of them life-threatening – fourteen times over. "They would just whittle away, trying to get the cancer," Barbara explained, "but leave my uterus and ovaries." In my thirty-plus years of gynecologic practice, I have neither treated nor heard of a single patient enduring fourteen surgeries for cancer or any other medical condition. I was stunned by the number and frequency of her surgeries: between one and three per year.

By 2012, three years after her cancer diagnosis, Barbara finally started asking for a hysterectomy. "I was just so tired of the surgeries," she said. "I just wanted the cancer gone." But both Barbara's husband and her surgeon wouldn't allow her a hysterectomy. Barbara paused and took a breath as she recalled these circumstances. "I was so frustrated by that. They would not let me decide."

Barbara's cancer recurred in 2014 and 2015, each recurrence requiring more surgery. "Finally, by 2016, seven years after my cancer was diagnosed – and after four years of my asking for a hysterectomy – my husband and my surgeon accepted that I might not have a baby, and they agreed to let me have a hysterectomy." Barbara's hysterectomy was her fourth laparotomy and last surgery, causing her to lose half of her bladder to

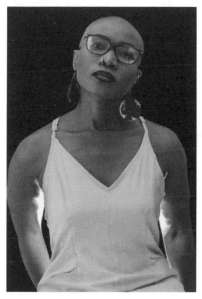

Figure 13.1 Barbara, whose husband left her after cervical cancer made her infertile

cancer. "It is such a relief to have my uterus gone and not worry about the cancer inside me," she said.

But Barbara's ordeal didn't end with the removal of her cancer and the cessation of yearly surgeries. After her hysterectomy, Barbara's husband left her. "I have been single," she said, "since 2017."

The Torment Continues

Barbara's suffering did not end with the cessation of yearly surgeries, the loss of possible parenthood, or the departure of her husband. The system in which that suffering occurred continued to torment her. "There is a huge stigma with having no children," she said. "The holier-than-thou people tell you, 'Maybe you are a sinner. You just did not pray enough.' The traditionalists have their own theories. And then there are just the normal, judgmental people. I have heard it all. Somehow, if

you do not have a baby, or do not have a uterus, you are an
outcast and are viewed as less than a woman."

> "There is a huge stigma with having no children,"
> she said. "The holier-than-thou people tell you,
> 'Maybe you are a sinner. You just did not pray
> enough.' The traditionalists have their own
> theories. And then there are just the normal,
> judgmental people. I have heard it all. Somehow,
> if you do not have a baby, or do not have a uterus,
> you are an outcast and are viewed as less than
> a woman."

In addition to her community maligning her for her lost uterus,
Barbara endured painful comments about having cervical cancer.
Because women in her culture are often blamed for illnesses associated with their reproductive organs, Barbara was held responsible for her own suffering, the worst kind of gaslighting. "People
are always looking for someone to blame. In fact, I have had people
in the medical profession tell me, 'You must have had sex before
the age of fifteen in order to get cervical cancer,'" Barbara said.
"There is a lot of body shaming in my country. People think if you
develop cervical cancer, you have been bewitched."

Barbara crystalized for me the formidable challenge of eradicating cervical cancer in communities or countries where patriarchy –
a system, either institutional or informal, in which men hold the
power and women are largely excluded from it – holds women in
unequal regard. Given the stigma around cervical cancer in her
country, Barbara said that it's nearly impossible to convince
women to support or seek prevention services.

Why Cash Alone Won't Cut It

The battle to provide cervical cancer prevention and treatment
for all cannot be solved solely with money. You can spend
millions or even billions to build clinics, buy colposcopy tools

and radiation equipment, attract proficient health care providers, and develop government policies that promote cervical cancer screening and prevention in lower-income countries or among marginalized populations in higher-income countries. Yet none of these purchases guarantees that a person with a cervix will get screened or receive the necessary treatment for cervical cancer.

Barbara had the access she needed: a ready Pap screening, a physician-husband who arranged her care, more surgeries than she could ever want. But the patriarchal social structures and community stigma around women and their bodies prolonged a terrible ordeal. Money might have bought her "care," but she was not cared for. She was tormented.

Patriarchy, sexual stigma, religious puritanism, fear and ignorance associated with women's bodies and reproductive organs, and the burden of women's unpaid work can all stop a woman from accessing cervical cancer care in the first place and make advocating for care and treatment a challenge few women have the energy or strength to take on. Add in the social vulnerabilities resulting from racial, gender, or status differences, and you have a long list of intangibles – things money cannot buy – impeding both cure and care. The end result? Women are made to suffer needlessly.

While it may seem challenging and even intimidating to tackle society's deep-seated and often emotion-laden beliefs, these mindsets represent the biggest barriers to change – the barriers we must address to save the hundreds of thousands of lives currently lost to cervical cancer every year.

Patriarchy Seeps in Everywhere

The silencing of Barbara's voice around her cervical cancer treatment demonstrates the pervasiveness of patriarchal culture. Patriarchal belief systems are entrenched over generations in many communities, regions, and countries around the world. Some patriarchal systems are formal and institutional; others

are informal and cultural. All hold women in lower regard than
men. While transforming systemic patriarchy is time-
consuming and complex, we need to be willing – at least in
the short term – to look the establishment in the eye, both at
home and abroad, and find creative, open-hearted, and collaborative ways to work within it. Time is of the essence if we really
want to eliminate cervical cancer.

From my North American vantage, it's easy to think of
patriarchy as something "over there." To say to myself,
"None of my friends or I would ever be in Barbara's position
culturally." It's easy to see patriarchy in the Taliban's ban on
education for girls or the kingdom of Saudi Arabia's ban on
women driving. But patriarchy doesn't just pose a barrier to
education in lower-income countries. Patriarchy seeps in
everywhere.

In higher-income countries, patriarchal culture seeps into
health care systems in subtle but insidious ways. Policies that
devalue medical care for women and their providers – and
thereby affect their access to cervical cancer prevention – are
the product of patriarchy. Consider the inequitable payment
system that government-funded or private insurance companies in the United States have designed for "male" versus
"female" medical procedures. Reimbursement standards have
long been shown to vastly favor surgeries or procedures performed on males, which means gynecologists are reimbursed at
lower rates for procedures than urologists performing equivalent procedures on males.

In a 2017 paper in *Gynecologic Oncology*, U.S. researchers
looked at payment inequity between 1997 and 2015 and
noted only minimal progress in payment equity over almost
two decades, with a *28-percent* higher rate of reimbursement
for 84 percent of male-based procedures compared with
equivalent female procedures.[1,2] A study published in 2021 in
Obstetrics and Gynecology found that while reimbursement for
procedures performed on females has gradually increased,
a discrepancy remained, with 58 percent of male-specific surgeries reimbursed at a higher rate than female-specific

procedures.[3,*] This persistent, gender-biased form of reimbursement discourages doctors from practicing "female" medicine and lowers the incentive to perform these procedures – creating a diminishing downward spiral on cervical cancer care. The study also looked at the committee that determined reimbursement rates and noted that, among its thirty voting members, only two were female. These findings reflect the way U.S. society values female health care and offer just one example of the male-dominated nature of U.S. medical care in which I practice. It's a stunning indictment of the embedded inequity we often overlook in this part of the world – a part of the world that prides itself on progressive thinking.

My patients frequently say they are thankful to have a female provider, a comment I've heard in all of the countries and continents I've offered gynecologic care. While I do not for one minute feel female providers should be the only ones conducting cervical cancer screening exams, the reality is they make many patients feel more comfortable and less vulnerable than they do with male providers. In the battle to eliminate cervical cancer, it makes sense to offer incentives to practicing female physicians so that more women seek HPV vaccines, screening exams, and other cancer-fighting procedures. Systems that discourage a ready supply of women practitioners are just another barrier to enticing persons with cervixes to seek lifesaving care.

---

* Medicare or insurance companies calculate reimbursement for medical procedures according to the relative value unit (RVU) they assign to procedures based on their complexity. This study compared the assigned RVUs and subsequent reimbursement offered per RVU for twelve roughly equivalent procedures performed for males and females. For example, the study looked at pelvic exenteration for prostate cancer in males compared with pelvic exenteration for cervical cancer in females, removal of the scrotum compared with removal of the vulva, drainage of an abscess on the penis compared with an abscess on the vulva, a scrotum biopsy compared with a vulvar biopsy and found that reimbursement per RVU for procedures performed only on females has only gradually improved in the past twenty years. However, a compensation gap persists for obstetrician/gynecologists performing surgeries on female bodies compared with urologists performing surgeries on male bodies, even though these surgeries have equally complex skill levels. The lower level of reimbursement observed for female surgeries has led researchers to believe in ongoing, perpetual gender bias within the medical community. R. M. Polan and E. L. Barber, "Reimbursement for Female-Specific Compared with Male-Specific Procedures over Time," *Obstet Gynecol* **138**, no. 6 (Dec 1 2021): 878–83. https://doi.org/10.1097/AOG.0000000000004599 www.ncbi.nlm.nih.gov/pubmed/34736273

Another manifestation of long-standing gender inequity is the well-documented pay-gap differences between female and male physicians, even within the same specialties. A 2022 study conducted by *Medscape*, one of the leading medical education platforms used by health care providers, found similar gender pay gaps among primary care physicians in the United Kingdom, Germany, France, United States, Brazil, and Mexico, with female doctors making 20 to 29 percent less than their male counterparts.[4] These gaps had only narrowed "slightly" in the past five years. Provider pay-gaps even exist in Canada where most physicians are paid set fees. A Canadian study authored by several Toronto-based physicians and published in *JAMA Surgery* in 2019 found Ontario female surgeons earned 24 percent less than their male peers, despite the province's fee-for-service payment model. The authors concluded that male specialists received more complex referrals than did female specialists.[5] By extension, male specialists tended to perform a greater number of technically difficult – and thereby more lucrative – surgical procedures than their female counterparts.

Equitable pay for female physicians and specialists holds direct implications for cervical cancer care: female providers attract and treat far more female patients. Higher pay for women providers means they're more likely to enter and remain in the system. In turn, female patients will have a greater number of sought-after, top-quality professionals to help them fight cervical cancer.

Squelching the Damage Caused by Gender Inequity

Patriarchal influences attack cervical cancer care in all kinds of ways. For Barbara, patriarchy came down like a sledgehammer, brutally demanding her body be carved up for the sake of sparing her fertility. For female reproductive-care physicians, patriarchy acts more like a paper cutter, whittling away at cervical cancer care by paying female doctors less for equivalent work and thereby discouraging them from staying in the medical system. In the quest to end cervical cancer, how do we stop the sledgehammer and blunt the paper cutter? What can be done to move beyond systems where men hold the power and possess the loudest voices and women's agency is squelched – either actively or insidiously? How do we address gender inequity's toll on cervical cancer elimination?

The answer to all of these questions is that despite the challenges of dismantling the patriarchy, we are seeing signs of improvement. To some degree, the WHO's recent commitment to cervical cancer elimination – and the worldwide attention it garners – reflects a new willingness to address inequities. Global change advocates are challenging traditions that previously allowed male-dominated governments to set policies and powers according to their own wish lists. Female-led decision-making bodies with influence and clout are combining with global power structures to raise women's voices and advocate for cervical cancer prevention. Women leaders are gaining momentum, their achievements visible across several continents, including those in North and South America, and Africa.

In Latin America, the Latin American Union against Cancer for Women has put female reproductive cancers on regional political agendas. In conjunction with the 2018 World Cancer Congress, the Union for International Cancer Control Regional Meeting for Latin America and the Caribbean hosted a forum that advocated for more attention and funding for women's cancer in Latin America.[6] In the wake of this event, the Latin American Union, a regional advocacy group representing cancer survivors and their families, promoted legislation and public policies toward reducing regional female cancers and cancer deaths. By magnifying women's voices in government, this group is working to overcome the patriarchal structures that prevent cervical cancer elimination from being at the top of countries' legislative and health agendas.

In Africa, a continent disproportionately plagued with cervical cancer deaths, another group of women is using its political clout to advocate for cervical cancer prevention and save women's lives. Led by thirty-seven wives of African presidents, the Organization of African First Ladies for Development aims to empower women and girls on the continent and offer them greater access to health care services. Traditionally focused on HIV care, the African First Ladies recently expanded its cervical cancer efforts by featuring HPV vaccination promotion in its four-year strategic plan.[7] "We have to offer communities a package of integrated approaches that include immunization, sexual and reproductive health, and rights and education," said First Lady of the Congo Antoinette Sassou Nguesso. First Lady of Côte d'Ivoire Dominique Ouattara has asked that this strategy focus on young African women's "equal and fair access to education and health care." Drawing on the strength of their voices, the members of the African First Ladies have shown how women can combat the all-pervasive patriarchy by influencing policy and priorities to keep a so-called woman's issue in the spotlight.

Kenya's County First Ladies Association, representing counties across the country, is following the African First Ladies' lead by advocating for greater HPV vaccine uptake, despite internal push-back. The County First Ladies were involved in the launch of Kenya's October 2019 HPV vaccine program, aimed at vaccinating more than 800,000 of the country's ten-year-old girls. But they faced strong opposition. Much of it came from a small group of doctors allied to the Kenya Catholic Doctors' Association, who swayed public opinion by sharing incorrect, fear-based information about the HPV vaccine and casting suspicion on the media's pro-vaccine message. They urged parents not to vaccinate their girls, concerned that HPV immunization was an invitation to early premarital sex.* As a result, only 30 percent of Kenya's

---

* A group of doctors allied to the Kenya Catholic Doctors' Association took its message to the media in 2019, urging parents not to allow their ten-year-old girls to receive the HPV vaccine. Among the association's myriad claims were doubts about vaccine safety and efficacy. They cited evidence, unbacked by science, from internet channels shown to be linked to anti-vaccination groups. They cautioned Kenyans that allowing the country's youth to receive vaccination against sexually transmitted HPV was tantamount to giving them free rein to engage in premarital sex. Instead, they urged the medical fraternity to focus on promoting abstinence among the unmarried and faithfulness within marriage to one sexual partner, and providing cervical cancer screening tests for sexually active women. "Kenyan Catholic Doctors Warn against Cervical Cancer Vaccination of Girls," *Catholic Philly*, updated Aug 22, 2019, accessed Jan 15, 2023. https://catholicphilly.com /2019/08/news/world-news/kenyan-catholic-doctors-warn-against-cervical-cancer-vaccination-of-girls/

targeted group of girls got vaccinated.[8] Nonetheless, the First Ladies remain undaunted, with a plan to continue advocating for widespread HPV vaccination among Kenyan girls. In a February 2020 online article, Dr. Phionah Atuhebwe, African regional immunization officer for the WHO, affirmed the County First Ladies' involvement in the campaign, writing that "women must work in the interests of fellow women."[9]

Also in Kenya, the organization Women 4 Cancer Early Detection & Treatment has been extensively raising awareness and advocating for cervical cancer prevention and treatment for the past three decades. Founded by three Kenyan women, Women 4 Cancer urged the Kenyan government to introduce the HPV vaccine. Benda Kithaka, the group's chair and cofounder, won the 2019 Distinguished Advocacy Award from the International Gynecologic Cancer Society for her work in education, advocacy, and policy development of cervical cancer prevention in Africa, an indication that a single group's persistence has the power to make a dent in the cervical cancer battle overseas.

Stigma Keeps Us Silent – and Silence Kills

Patriarchy doesn't just exist within institutions and systems. One of its most insidious features is the stigma it fosters around women's bodies and sexuality, a stigma often born of traditional or religious notions of female chastity and purity. Stigma promises relational, social, even spiritual punishment – all powerful incentives for a killer cancer to flourish.

Barbara talked about the acute sense of stigma she endured by having and being treated for cervical cancer. A medical professional told her it was "her fault" she had the disease, that she "must have had sex before the age of fifteen." Virtually every cervical cancer survivor I spoke with for this book described suffering from the stigma associated with the disease. Some of these shame-inducing comments, such as those Barbara heard, came from medical providers;

others came from friends or family who appeared ill informed about the causes of cervical cancer or steeped in patriarchal beliefs about cervical cancer sufferers acquiring the disease because they'd failed to adhere to cultural norms. And I've had many U.S. or international patients reporting being shamed with comments like "oh, you must have gotten cervical cancer from sex with too many partners," or "gosh – I thought you only got cervical cancer if you had other sexually transmitted infections too." Shaming does not have to come from men; women can be the torch bearers for misogyny – making it vital to target both sexes in educational campaigns about cervical cancer.

Blaming women for acquiring cervical cancer can be seen as a defense mechanism. Cervical cancer is scary. One way a woman can feel less scared is to focus on behavior as a way to rationalize the source of cervical cancer. This insidious form of "othering" allows a woman to separate herself from "the woman who brought it on herself through too many sexual partners or having sex at a young age." But this kind of thinking only fosters the stigma of cervical cancer, adding to the hurt and isolation a woman like Barbara endured even while undergoing treatment for her disease. "Blame culture" singles out cervical cancer patients and compounds their suffering.

Blaming women for acquiring cervical cancer can be seen as a defense mechanism. Cervical cancer is scary. One way a woman can feel less scared is to focus on behavior as a way to rationalize the source of cervical cancer.

The anatomy of cervical cancer also contributes to its stigma. The cervix sits at the top of the vagina, and neither the cervix nor the vagina is an anatomical structure that people talk about openly. For some, the vagina is even considered "dirty" – just look at the number of commercial products promising to "clean" it. An entire industry has been built on promoting unnecessary and even harmful feminine hygiene products for a body part that needs no washing at all! I've met patients in Texas, Nicaragua, and Kenya who were falsely taught that they needed to clean their genital tracts and did so either by cutting into their hard-earned, household budget or by relying on potentially harmful, self-made cleaning products. When I worked in Kenya, some of my female patients reported using bleach powder to clean their vaginas. This is where we start to see the physical harm associated with stigma. Bleach powder and other "cleaning" products cause defects in the protective layers of the vaginal lining, leading to small ulcers, which leave users even more likely to contract viruses like HIV.[10,11] Talk about a tragic irony: a woman cleaning her "dirty" parts is made even more vulnerable to stigma, shame, and disease. Until we start talking openly about our misguided thinking about female reproductive health – and what we can do to alter it – stigma and silence will continue to kill.

Women Strike Back

The desire to move beyond the stigma associated with cervical cancer is the reason so many women tell me they're motivated to become cervical cancer advocates. These survivors want to live without the added burden of stigma. By becoming cervical cancer champions, they take their power back, rejecting stigma's power to isolate and humiliate.

After her terrible journey with cervical cancer "care" in the patriarchy, Barbara channeled her counseling expertise into cervical cancer advocacy, founding Bold Dialogue, an organization that "aims to empower, inspire and guide women to become the best versions of themselves." She developed a coaching practice that supports women, and she has written books and blogs for cervical cancer education, inspiring other women to overcome challenges within male-dominated cultural and value systems. Barbara is using her gifts in creative ways and with great courage.

She's taking on harmful patriarchal structures simply by refusing to let them silence her.

And then there's Carol, who underwent life-changing pelvic exenteration surgery and now lives with a urostomy and a colostomy. As she faced traumatic physical disfigurement, Carol endured comments from others implying that she could have avoided her cancer, that she'd brought misfortune on herself. This is "othering" and blaming at its worst. As Carol said to me, what these women don't know is that they, like over 80 percent of all sexually active people, will eventually get HPV. "Unfortunately for me," Carol pointed out, "the HPV persisted." Until we're ready to turn blame on its head and let it morph into social responsibility, cervical cancer sufferers will be doubly tortured – by their disease and by others' ignorant thinking about it. Carol was not to blame. She was simply unfortunate. And she refuses to hide and take the blame for what happened to her. Carol talks openly about cervical cancer and its toll on her life and body, boldly referring to her unique anatomy as a "barbie butt," and owning her experience with humor and resiliency (Figure 13.2). In fact, just by coming forward and allowing their stories to be featured in this book, women like Carol and Barbara – and all the other amazing women I spoke with – are translating their shame into bravery: passionate about educating others about the role of HPV in cervical cancer and advocating for disease prevention.

As long as women feel ashamed of or ill-attuned to their bodies' needs, they cannot care for themselves properly, regardless of their access to care. Talking openly about HPV, cervical cancer screening, and women's anatomy, and educating each other about disease prevention dismantles the stigma and shame sur-rounding cervical cancer. As women's familiarity with and accept-ance of their bodies grows, so does their power. When we come together and support each other as women – in solidarity for the bodies we're given, affected by cervical cancer or not – we are taking concrete steps to overcome the stigma that discourages us from trying to prevent cervical cancer in the first place.

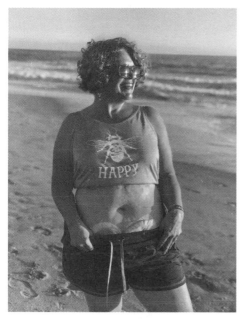

Figure 13.2 Carol, who underwent pelvic exenteration surgery against cervical cancer

The Burden of Unpaid Work

Societies devalue women in one of the most basic and universal ways by asking them to assume the greater burden of unpaid work. Around the world, women do a disproportionate share of the caretaking that supports families and communities – and they mostly do so for free. Raising children; caring for parents; upholding organizations that support schools, churches, temples, mosques, and synagogues; sustaining arts and cultural organizations that enrich society as a whole – all of these activities comprise the vastly undercompensated or uncompensated purview of women. In lower-income countries, women's duties include hours and hours every day spent gathering firewood and clean water, cooking, cleaning, farming, and child-rearing. The types and contribution levels of unpaid work may vary among individuals – based on where they live, their incomes, and their social status – but women bearing the brunt of these expectations does not vary. Study after study has documented the burden of unpaid work on women's physical well-being, parenting, professional capacities, and overall mental health.[12-17] The toll of unpaid work remains disturbingly consistent from one part of the world to another.

The burden of unpaid labor can leave little time and much less energy for what is often referred to as "self-care." But self-care as it relates to women's health is not optional – it is medically essential. Remember Kim from Chapter 8, who was diagnosed with cervical cancer after allowing many years to pass between Pap smears. A busy professional with eight children and a commitment to care for others, including her friend Elvia's community in Haiti, Kim had forgotten – and certainly her community never reinforced – that reproductive care is a necessity. When women's unpaid labor gets in the way of health care, including cervical cancer prevention measures, labor's true cost is unacceptable.

The toll of unpaid labor might translate into working women being unable to leave their paid jobs or care of elderly relatives or young children in order to see a doctor. For others, the burden can look like a woman choosing between feeding her family or caring for her body. Women wear this iron mantle of unpaid work, ubiquitous across countries and cultures, like a ball and chain against the freedom, mobility, and support they need to be able to care for themselves.

Getting One Half of the World to Lift Up the Other

In *The Moment of Lift* (Flatiron Books, 2019), Melinda Gates describes the built-in trap for women opposing the inequitable burden of unpaid work. The imbalanced load on women to complete household chores and oversee childcare, she writes, cannot be addressed without acknowledging the underlying gender biases behind how that work is assigned. The free labor one half of the population supplies to benefit the other half offers little motivation for changing the arrangement.

According to a 2020 Oxfam report on global income inequality, the monetary value of unpaid work for women fifteen and over equals at least $10.8 trillion USD every year, an appraisal the authors described as "three times the size of the world's tech industry."[14] But asking the world to equate women's unpaid work with the worth of the tech industry – much less declare it three times more valuable – sounds like an elusive goal.

What is not elusive is the effect of unpaid work on women's health care needs. In my thirty years as a gynecologist, if I counted the number of persons with cervixes I've seen delay their screening appointments for being "just too busy" or "unable to get away," and added to that the women in this book who said the same thing and ended up having cancer, would women have suffered "enough" to justify putting self-care at the top of their lists? How many women need to acquire a preventable cancer because unpaid work stopped them from getting a simple medical exam before the world says, "Enough"?

From a purely biological perspective, men contribute to cervical cancer's deadly rampage when they carry and share HPV with their sexual partners. Men also stand to lose when the women in their lives, their communities, and their countries die of cervical cancer. As Melinda Gates so astutely observes, a steady flow of free labor may undermine the desires of its beneficiaries to upend the status quo. At the very least, however, can we not call on men who have a vested interest in the health of women who serve them? When women get sick or die, who will then care for their children, their parents, their neighbors, their communities? Men have a lot to gain from eliminating cervical cancer and keeping women alive.

Of course, I want more than that. I want men to join the fight to transform patriarchal norms and laws and support women in leadership positions. I want them to empower women to make important decisions about their own health care. I want them to support and advocate for their mothers, sisters, wives, and daughters because they have intrinsic human value. But as cervical cancer rates rise around the world, I'll settle for a cause largely led by female cervical cancer sufferers and survivors – and organizations acting on behalf of a global ethos of social responsibility – until the pressure becomes too much for the rest of us to bear.

But while we continue to live under a patriarchal social order, I want each man to make sure all of the women in his life get cervical cancer screening. I want fathers to get their daughters vaccinated against HPV. And I want men to speak out about their beliefs that health care for women is a right. Even as they begin to question their roles and inspire change around the structures that hold all of us down, we need men to join a fight now that benefits us all.

A License to Be Licentious – or a License to Live?

Puritanical thinking – the notion that chastity precludes HPV vaccination – represents another intangible barrier to cervical cancer prevention. Social scientists often attribute this thinking to patriarchal societies that favor virginal women.

In the United States, conservative religious groups in particular are uncomfortable with vaccinating children against a sexually transmitted infection. They have objected to the introduction of the HPV vaccination and discouraged its use by invoking the specter of sexual promiscuity. The fact that the vaccine was originally described as a tool for preventing a sexually transmitted infection rather than for cancer prevention has only added to parents' fears and hampered vaccination uptake in our country for years.

But studies conducted over the past fifteen years in both higher- and lower-income countries have failed to demonstrate any correlation between the HPV vaccine and earlier or more frequent engagement in sex. In the United States, a study of sexual behaviors in 700,000 adolescents from 2001 to 2015 found no sexual behavioral changes related to HPV education.[18] A different team of U.S. investigators found HPV vaccination had no effect on sexual activity among youth entering college.[19] A U.S. study of more than 20,000 adolescents between 2005 and 2010 also found no relation between HPV vaccination and the acquisition of sexually transmitted infections.[20]

Studies of this kind are not limited to the United States. In Uganda, researchers compared sexual activity in 400 adolescent females in 2014 and found no link between early sexual activity and those who'd benefited from receiving the HPV vaccine.[21] A 2020 study in Brazil found HPV vaccination did not increase sexual activity.[22] In Australia, the messaging is clear: HPV vaccination does not change sexual activity in adolescents.[23] Yet, the fear-based belief that HPV vaccination influences an adolescent's decisions about sex interferes with its uptake. The real fear should be about unvaccinated girls getting cervical cancer as adults.

Medical associations, such as the American Academy of Pediatrics and the Society of Gynecologic Oncology, and public health agencies, such as the CDC and the WHO, have altered the prevention of sexually transmitted infections message to promoting HPV vaccination for cancer prevention. As a result, uptake has gradually improved in countries like the United States, despite the original reluctance. In my medical practice, I am seeing growing acceptance of the vaccine. But whenever I talk about the vaccine with parents of teens, they raise the issue of early involvement in sex, and I share the reassuring findings that HPV vaccination does not confer license to have sex. This kind of "talking back" to the lie that vaccination promotes promiscuity, that cervical cancer is the result of sexual licentiousness, is something each one of us can engage in – free of charge.

No More "Speculum Surprises"

As I said earlier, patriarchy seeps in everywhere. The stigma around women's bodies and women's sexuality can lodge deep in their psyches, regardless of personal beliefs about equality and individual worth. This stigma, as well as a natural aversion to pelvic exams, hinders women from overcoming their resistance to screening, despite its critical role in prevention.

Having a speculum examination is a moment of true vulnerability. The words that a medical provider frequently offers – "just relax, let your knees fall apart, and try to make the muscles of your vagina soft" – sound ludicrous to any person with a cervix, stripped bare and lying down on an exam table. If a woman is uncomfortable with her body or somehow considers it "dirty," a pelvic exam can be a terrible invasion of privacy. The feeling of vulnerability during a pelvic exam is compounded for women who have been sexually assaulted. A U.S. study of 1,500 women sexually assaulted as children showed that they were significantly less likely to be up to date on their screening exams.[24] Given that studies of violence against women suggest as many as one in six[25] have been sexually assaulted, it is easy to understand why fear and anxiety keep so many women away from cervical cancer screening.

Overcoming women's aversion to screening takes more than money – it requires genuine compassion. Tamika Felder, founder of the international cervical cancer advocacy group Cervivor, said the medical community needed to better prepare women for their first pelvic examinations. "Providers do not give women an idea of what it is about or why it is important," she said. "And that speculum – well, it just surprises you." When providers approach women with gentle awareness and concern, they can make adjustments to help them "stay in the stirrups" and come back without fear.

Fewer medical "surprises" of the kind Tamika Felder refers to may be one way to establish a woman's lifelong pattern for timely cervical cancer screening – providing she can tackle other barriers to accessing these tests. Rather than being viewed as an unpleasant hurdle, speculum-based screening can be promoted as an important part of a woman taking care of herself and feeling empowered to make proactive decisions around her own health.

Talk, Talk, Talk

Money can't take down patriarchal or religious attitudes about sex, women, their bodies, or their worth. To change any cultural narrative, we're better off naming the prejudices associated with it and countering those beliefs with knowledge, sound reasoning, and conviction. We succeed by lifting up and amplifying women's voices along the way. Every woman I interviewed for this book spoke with not only great courage but also candor. Their stories are powerful because they spoke unsparingly, in full ownership of their experiences and unwilling to silence any part of them. When we talk about our bodies freely with other persons with cervixes, we take part in shifting the larger conversation. Rather than criticizing how women handle their reproductive health, we harness the power of talk to enlighten and educate the world about cervical cancer.

When women talk openly about their pelvic exam or Pap smear experiences or even their cervical cancer treatment, other women are more likely to get screened or have their children vaccinated. Women talking openly about what it's like to survive cancer – and the suffering and courage they call upon daily to move forward – can offer strength to women facing the same ordeal. Their words can inspire women to avoid the same fate by getting screened. Women talking openly about their vaginas and their cervixes can normalize those body parts, denying stigma its insidious power. Women talking openly about just how common HPV is can make a sexually transmitted virus a fact of life rather than a source of shame. Women talking openly about the miracle of the HPV vaccine can inspire parents to have their children vaccinated without fear. Let's talk so much and so openly about cervical cancer prevention that it becomes as easy to discuss as breast cancer prevention – or any other disease, for that matter, that's become part of an easy public conversation.

And while women are talking to other women, let's bring the men along. Let's talk to men about their role in HPV transmission, assuring men know that the virus is sexually transmitted. Let's talk to them about the benefit of their daughters getting HPV vaccinations. Let's talk to them about the importance of the women in their lives getting screened. Let's talk with men about the gift that cervical cancer prevention is to them, their children, and society for its power to keep women healthy. Let's recruit the men we talk to so they can talk with other men. Let's talk so much that we engender male champions for cervical cancer prevention – ready and willing to join the throngs of women acting as witnesses to each other. Money cannot buy any of this. Money cannot bring down the wall of patriarchy. Money cannot release women from social expectations or free men from the prison it holds them in as well. Even Barbara's husband suffered his own ordeal: by submitting to the belief that her fertility mattered more than her overall health, he lost an amazing woman. Let's crush the power of stigma by breaking the silence and supporting desensitization – referring casually to words formerly deemed "below-the-belt": *vagina*, *cervix*, *HPV*. Let's lessen the weight of unpaid work, recognizing that it sits on the backs of women, creating loads so heavy it precludes them from seeking the health care they need and deserve.

In the fight against cervical cancer, money can buy a lot. But it cannot take down the forbidding wall of patriarchy, stigma, inequality, religious puritanism, fear, and ignorance. For that, we need to talk. We need honesty, candor, vulnerability, courage. Money cannot buy the power of women talking to women, women talking to men, citizens talking to their governments, or survivors talking to the world. Money cannot buy the transformation that happens when, as we talk, we listen. One brick at a time, let's knock down that wall, which prevents hundreds of thousands of women from reaching out for what they need to prevent the tragedy that is cervical cancer.

Part Four
Getting to Enough

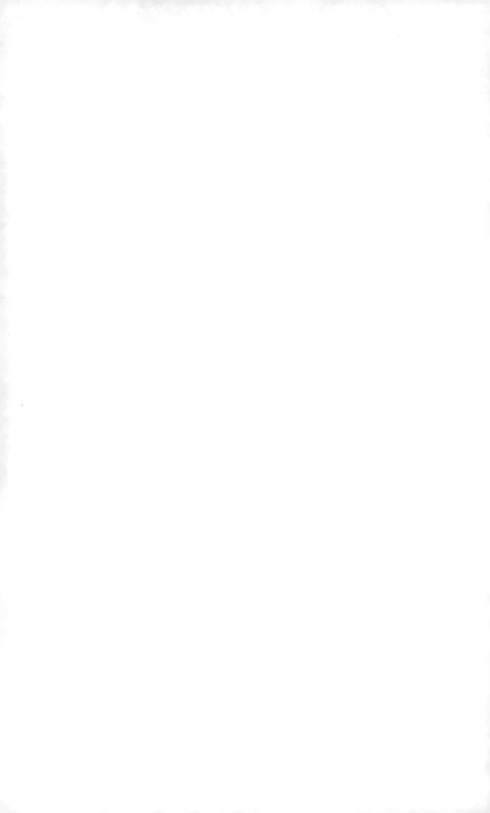

14 A SEA CHANGE STARTS WITH A RIPPLE

In reading about the epic challenges in defeating cervical cancer, are you starting to feel the sense of helplessness I did when I first met Mama dying on an exam table? The knowledge that prompted this cry in the dark: "Can't I help?" Or this haunting refrain from the powerless: "Can any of us help any of these women? Ever? At all?"

These questions are understandable – reasonable, even. Sometimes I ask myself how 194 member countries of the World Health Organization (WHO), faced with an endless range of peak-sized challenges, committed to the future elimination of this rapacious disease. How did they have the courage to sign on? Think about the odds stacked against them: 90 percent of those who die of cervical cancer every year live in countries offering one oncologist for a thousand people or one radiation machine to serve 5 million; many struggle to provide even basic health care or blood for transfusions in surgery; their national health budgets are beyond meager and often beholden to the help of nongovernmental organizations (NGOs); their citizens labor under deep stigma around women's reproductive systems; and their women struggle to find the time, energy, or money to even seek care for themselves. If the world needs to turn all of that around to save these women, where will the world even start?

Throughout this book, I've said this effort will take a "sea change." I am talking about a profound transformation in political will around women's health and, frankly, a recognition of women's value to society – a value extended to persons with cervixes who experience marginalization by race, orientation, ethnicity, income, or geography. As is often the case with any momentous shift concerning human rights, this sea change of efforts will begin with ripples, tiny circles created by small stones that travel outward. If we ever hope to see the end of more than 340,000 preventable deaths a year, it's going to take stone after stone, ripple after ripple, to make waves.

To reach the shores that lie ahead of eliminating cervical cancer altogether.

A few years ago in Zambia, Karen Nakawala, a local radio and television personality there, tossed one of those pebbles in the water.

From Reluctant Advocate to Stone-Thrower

Talking with Karen felt instantly easy to me. Even over Zoom from her home office in the capital city of Lusaka, her voice was as welcoming and smooth as butter sliding onto warm bread. I was struck by her infectious, hearty smile, and her alert and expressive brown eyes. It was hard to believe that just seventeen months before our conversation, she was fighting for her life. Karen was diagnosed with Stage 2B cancer of the cervix at forty-five years old. She described herself as overly confident she would never face a disease like cervical cancer.

"I was one of those women who never went for screening. I was healthy, eating well, exercising, and just did not think it would happen to me." The only reason she got screened was to appease her friend, a gynecologist, who'd been pestering her to come for an appointment. She finally relented. "My gynecologist took one look at my cervix, and right away asked me if I was feeling okay, if I had any pain or bleeding," Karen recalled. "I had been having dull back pain, but I thought it was from wearing high heels too much. And, I'd had a little bleeding between periods, but I thought that was because I was getting close to menopause."

A week later, Karen received her diagnosis. "I felt like I was in an ice cube when I heard the word 'cancer,'" she said. "I moved into this robotic state. I immediately started seeing myself as dead, and the first thing I wondered was who would take care of my ten- and twenty-four-year-old girls."

Two weeks later, Karen started radiation therapy augmented by chemotherapy, and at the end of twenty-three external radiation treatments, she received four brachytherapy treatments. In retrospect, she felt fortunate. "Usually, it can take months in Zambia to get started with radiation treatment."

But, like every other patient in Zambia, Karen faced the stigma associated with cervical cancer. She had a hard time telling anyone about her diagnosis, including her partner. "I felt he would run away from me. But actually, he was very supportive, and I don't think I could have gone through this without him." Karen continued working while she received her radiation treatments. "I did not want anyone to know I was sick." And yet, although Karen had shared her diagnosis with only her partner and a few close friends, somehow the news leaked onto Facebook. Because of her public profile, Karen quickly found strangers approaching her on social media.

"That triggered something in me," she said. "I started thinking, 'You know, I can actually do something about it.' My partner also encouraged me to come forward . . . I guess you could say I became a reluctant advocate." During her treatment, Karen had begun to realize the dearth of information about cervical cancer in her country. "In fact, three-fourths of the women who were getting brachytherapy for cervical cancer with me had no idea what cervical cancer was. One woman from a rural area of Zambia told me she was bewitched . . . her daughter had to go get her in her rural village and bring her to Lusaka to get treatment, because the woman did not believe in cancer." Karen suggested that Zambian lack of awareness about cervical cancer stems from a general avoidance of reproductive health problems. "Any disease 'below the belt' is taboo and cannot be talked about, especially in public. Many women suffer and die in silence."

That morbid silence troubled Karen. "I did some soul-searching," she said. "I realized it took a long time in Zambia for the country to begin talking about HIV freely, like in churches, or just among family or friends. But, when we did start talking about HIV, people started getting tested and treated, couples went together for testing, and things got better."

This profound shift in thinking about HIV made Karen wonder if people could change their minds about a similarly destructive disease. It inspired her to ask herself a life-changing question: "What if we started talking about cervical cancer?"

Karen created a Facebook group called Teal Sisters, hoping to promote safe and private discussions about cervical cancer and encourage cervical vaccination and screening. It was a hit. "Within just a few days," she remembered, "hundreds of women joined. In fact, within two weeks, I got an invitation from the First Lady of Zambia to speak on cervical cancer. And now we have people not just from Zambia, but also from neighboring African countries, even from the United States, who are part of our Facebook group."

Teal Sisters quickly evolved beyond discussions among survivors to an advocacy platform for cervical cancer screening. "Our strategy was to get women to go together in groups for screening," Karen said. "Go with your friends, talk to them about cervical cancer, and bring them with you, together, so you can support each other through this new experience." Karen also hoped to address a general lack of understanding in Zambia about the value of the HPV vaccine, particularly among hesitant parents. "People don't know that the vaccine will help prevent HPV as children grow and become sexually active."

Since Karen started Teal Sisters, more than 100,000 Zambian women have joined the Facebook group, and they have started a Teal Sisters Foundation to raise money in support of cervical cancer prevention and disease sufferers. Their efforts have paid for screening services for women in prison and treatment for those traveling to Lusaka for radiation. The Teal Sisters also works directly with the Zambian health ministry to coordinate awareness-raising events in conjunction with planned screening services at local health facilities. The group generates increased demand for these services through distribution of ministry-approved education materials about the importance of cervical cancer prevention, and by encouraging local information-sharing about the disease. The Teal Sisters also uses performance art to directly engage with each community to build trust and promote further discussion. These activities feature local actors demonstrating the cervical screening process and teaching audiences directly about cervical cancer through drama, dance, and song. "We also take advantage of large gatherings, such as traditional marriage ceremonies, church gatherings, and women's conferences to speak about cervical cancer," Karen said. Their initiatives include visiting companies that employ large female workforces. Grassroots efforts like those provided by the Teal Sisters are one of the reasons the country now leads the way in sub-Saharan Africa for cervical screening rates.[1]

Teal Sisters' willingness to champion survivors allows members to speak directly and passionately about their experiences with cervical cancer, activities that Karen said strike a chord among communities looking for honesty and personal connection. Karen worked in partnership with the WHO during its preparation to launch the cervical cancer elimination strategy, telling her story via video where it was broadcast around the globe. She admitted her media background might have made it easier for her to talk about her experience. "But it is still hard to tell a personal story," she said.

Telling one's story is hard. I encountered that truth over and over as I spoke with survivors for this book. None of them found it easy to relive what they'd been through. But all of them spoke to me because they passionately wanted to help other women avoid the suffering they'd endured. Each knew her voice was uniquely powerful. Karen attributes Teal Sisters' success to the power of women sharing stories. "Survivors are the best people to tell the story of preventing and treating cervical cancer. If anyone is going to be believed, it has to come from someone who has walked that road."

> *"Survivors are the best people to tell the story of preventing and treating cervical cancer. If anyone is going to be believed, it has to come from someone who has walked that road."*

Pick Up a Pebble; Survivors Can't Do This Alone

Life handed Karen what many of us would consider a heavy stone: a diagnosis of cervical cancer and the fear, uncertainty, and stigma that comes with it (Figure 14.1). But Karen took that stone and tossed it back into the world, using her platform to share her story and gather others to do the same – with powerful implications. The ripples of her story and those of thousands of other Teal Sisters are changing the landscape of public attitudes about cervical cancer in Zambia, and changing the physical landscape with improved infrastructure at the same time. Zambia now has one of the best screening programs in sub-Saharan Africa, innovatively using nurses to administer it, often in conjunction with more established HIV clinics. Those efforts – combined with honesty, activism, and advocacy from the Teal Sisters – are making waves.

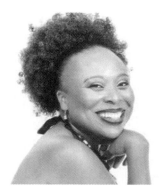

Figure 14.1 Karen Nakawala, founder of the Teal Sisters in Zambia

But survivors cannot and should not bear this burden alone. To take down cervical cancer will require many, many pebbles, and more and more ripples. Karen speaks passionately about the need for men's support and is grateful her partner has started speaking out to other men about cervical cancer. "Men here do not want women to get screened. They think, 'The vagina is my property. I paid for it. The vagina is mine,'" she pointed out. "I have realized you cannot win this fight against cervical cancer without the men." And so, Teal Sisters has been working closely with husbands, fathers, and sons. "We've been letting them know they should be the ones to save their wives by allowing them to get screened, and they should be the ones to take their children to get vaccinated." Karen draws on Zambia's successful campaigns against the spread of HIV. "I have seen males now go with women together for HIV screening so they can learn how to protect each other. We can do that teaching with cervical cancer prevention."

"I have realized you cannot win this fight against cervical cancer without the men."

Cape Town gynecologic oncologist Dr. Lynette Denny also sees the power of grassroots activism – the way it enfolds whole communities in promoting preventative care. To increase demand for and uptake of screening in their clinic, these change advocates relied on local support from traditional healers, chiefs, churches, and other groups to explain the benefits of screening and improve trust between the clinic and the community. Seeking to meet others "on the ground," the clinic sponsored a health festival, and its staff toured the township with singing and celebratory music, including an original praise song that celebrated reproduction and the "beauty of the vagina." Dr. Denny was clear that the benefits of this event came not from her own efforts, but those of the local community, who embraced, normalized, even celebrated reproductive health. Dr. Denny said local women have begun recognizing, accepting, and, in turn, accessing screening services, citing this "on-the-ground" movement as a critical step toward starting a cervical cancer screening program in Cape Town.

Grassroots advocacy is accelerated when larger organizations with deep pockets and wide influence are there to fund and support it, much the way a heavier rock makes a bigger splash – a larger ripple expanding wide into the distance. In Rwanda, HPV vaccination rates are an astonishing 95 percent, owing, in part, to cooperation between the Rwandan government, Gavi, and Girl Effect, a nonprofit group based in the United Kingdom.[2] Girl Effect's use of multiple platforms – a magazine, radio drama and talk show, moderated online communities, and brand ambassadors – allowed the group's message to reach 80 percent of Rwandan girls.

Based in the United States, the Global Initiative Against HPV and Cervical Cancer (GIAHC) is another "heavy rock." It relies on influence, partnerships, and coalitions for advocacy, education, training, and awareness building toward eliminating cervical cancer. GIAHC used its institutional power to boost one woman's voice and story in producing the acclaimed documentary, *Lady Ganga: Nilza's Story*. The film chronicles the journey of cervical cancer sufferer Michele Baldwin, who paddle-boarded 700 miles of the Ganges River during the last months of her life to bring awareness to the disease. The movie had 40,000 YouTube views in its first three years and is now being dubbed into Hindi to reach more people in India. The making of the film shows an organization with influence and reach working in partnership with one strong, determined woman, elevating her voice and shining a light on her personal battle for the benefit of other women.

Advocates like Karen and Michele have unique power, their stories and experiences rippling forcefully and farther, reaching more women, more powerfully. Karen's ripple became the 100,000-member wave that is Teal Sisters, and Michele's ripple surged across an entire continent, filmed for thousands more to see. Ripples like these are integral to the fight against cervical cancer: in partnership with influential organizations, they can stir up turbulent waters, calling attention to the preventable suffering or death of hundreds of thousands of women. At the same time, as Karen told me, advocacy goes beyond raising awareness: it must include a dramatic push for access to cervical cancer prevention, which cannot happen without a society's widespread support. The ripples must become waves, breaking across the shores of research, medicine, and funding platforms of every kind. Without sustained courage and innovation – confined to the gentle ripples of pebbles here and there – the WHO's commitment to eliminate cervical cancer will never surge far or fast enough to vanquish the disease for good.

The Tidal Wave: Innovations in Vaccination

Around the world, researchers are hefting larger and larger stones that – pitched into the pond of cervical cancer – create exciting ripples of hope, even tidal waves. One such wave is a development in the area of HPV vaccination, specifically around dosage. Research trials are underway in Costa Rica, Tanzania, and Kenya to see if just one – rather than the currently recommended two doses – of the HPV vaccine will suffice, thanks to funding by the National Cancer Institute and the Bill & Melinda Gates Foundation, and the collaboration of the University of Nairobi, the University of Washington, the National Cancer Institute, and the London School of Tropical Medicine. A one-dose vaccine regimen would be easier to administer, alleviate the complications of tracking and monitoring for the second dose, and – perhaps most significantly – cut the current cost in half while potentially doubling supply. From a global perspective, single-dose vaccination would immediately counter worldwide vaccine shortages, and almost surely make the vaccine more widely available to marginalized and impoverished populations around the world.

The great news is that the 2022 results from the Kenya trial showed that a single dose of HPV vaccine was as effective as two or three doses in preventing the HPV infections that lead to cervical cancer.[3] Based on these studies, the WHO's Strategic Advisory Group of Experts on Immunization (SAGE) voted to recommend a single dose of HPV vaccine for anyone between nine and fourteen. Imagine the implications for persons with cervixes: just a single shot can prevent 90 percent of cervical cancer.* A tidal wave, indeed.

Another wave gathering strength comes from three new HPV vaccines on trial in India and China that could alleviate the current shortage. According to a recent WHO report, these vaccines (China is testing two of them) could offer a fivefold supply increase over the next ten years.[4] In 2021, the WHO provided its "prequalification" stamp of approval for Cecolin®, one of the Chinese vaccines.[5] These additional vaccine options and the new, one-dose vaccination option represent exciting "swells" in the area of HPV prevention – swells being met by other ripples from the cervical cancer elimination effort.[6]

Expanding the Ripples through Screening Innovations

In response to the WHO's updated 2021 screening and treatment recommendations for cervical cancer prevention, the field of screening provides a surge of hope for countries eager to adopt HPV-DNA testing. These developments are consistent with the WHO's preference for increasingly accurate HPV-DNA testing over any other testing strategy.

Besides being a better predictor of pre-cancer than VIA or Pap smears alone, the HPV-DNA test is run by machines, and is less subject to human error. A negative HPV-DNA test result offers a 99 percent likelihood cervical cancer will not develop within five years, making these tests a far better option against keeping up with regular VIA or Pap screening. Another substantial benefit to HPV screening is vaginal swab collection. The ease of testing offers greater flexibility around how, when, and where

---

* The nonavalent HPV vaccine protects against 90 percent of cervical cancer, and the quadrivalent and bivalent vaccines protect against 70 percent of cervical cancer.
  A. Yusupov, D. Popovsky, L. Mahmood, et al., "The Nonavalent Vaccine: A Review of High-Risk HPVs and a Plea to the CDC," *Am J Stem Cells* **8**, no. 3 (2019): 52–64.
  www.ncbi.nlm.nih.gov/pubmed/31976155

it's administered. Patients can attend a clinic and conduct the HPV-DNA test collection themselves, with no need for traditional pelvic examinations or standard Pap testing equipment – such as exam tables or speculums – or even the extra paid provider time for these services. Or, patients can collect these swabs in the privacy of their own homes.

HPV-DNA testing is not only more accurate than Pap testing, but it can also alleviate screening pressures and wait times and potentially offer patients easier access to this cancer-prevention step. HPV-DNA tests can also be provided in any standard medical clinic, diminishing patients' concerns about the stigma of going to an HIV clinic for screening. What's more, clinics can readily convert "PCR-detecting machines" that NGOs and higher-income governments distributed worldwide during the height of the COVID-19 pandemic into HPV-DNA testing devices. Given their innumerable advantages, HPV-DNA tests are currently considered the "Screen and Treat" method of choice against cervical cancer.

The only drawback with HPV-DNA testing, however, is price – still a hurdle in many regions of the world. While multiple continents are researching more affordable versions, the cheapest available HPV-DNA tests are about $15 USD apiece, to say nothing of the several-thousand-dollar price tag for the machines required to process them.* Additional impediments associated with these tests include the hard-to-obtain chemicals to conduct them, along with the scarcity of affordable service contracts to maintain the testing machines. As a result, HPV-DNA testing is beyond the range of many health care budgets in lower-income countries, making it a rare cervical cancer prevention option for the regions of the world that need it most.

For countries forced to rely on less effective VIA testing, however, one ripple of innovation shows promise. Unlike

---

* The development of true "point-of-care" tests that can be processed immediately, without requiring a lot of equipment or time (similar to a pregnancy test or a COVID-19 nasal swab test) will be hugely helpful to bringing HPV-DNA testing to lower-income countries. Y. N. Flores, D. M. Bishai, A. Lorincz, *et al.*, "HPV Testing for Cervical Cancer Screening Appears More Cost-Effective Than Papanicolau Cytology in Mexico," *Cancer Causes Control* **22**, no. 2 (Feb 2011): 261–72. https://doi.org/10.1007/s10552-010-9694-3 www.ncbi.nlm.nih.gov/pubmed/21170578

a machine-read HPV-DNA test, a VIA test requires a human provider to visually assess the cervix. Because untrained observers can confuse cancer with inflammation from common conditions like cervical infections or vaginal yeast infections, VIA providers require ongoing, expert training and supervision. Researchers have been exploring the use of artificial intelligence in interpreting VIA findings as a means of lessening the human-error factor. This rapidly evolving technique, automated visual evaluation (AVE), uses a computer algorithm to evaluate digital images of a cervix from a cell phone or handheld, portable colposcope. The algorithm relies on artificial intelligence and machine-learning to detect early cellular changes signaling cancer. Current AVE trials, sponsored by the National Cancer Institute, are underway in nine countries with hoped-for results by 2024.[7,8] Once trials are completed, this automated technology would require less rigorous supervision and quality monitoring, be easier to use than VIA, and reduce the cost of VIA training, thus addressing a key bottleneck in screening.

Innovation around the delivery of screening programs is also having dramatic impact. With the support of PEPFAR (the U.S. President's Emergency Plan for AIDS Relief), twelve African countries – including Botswana, Namibia, Malawi, and Mozambique, along with eight others – have aligned HIV care with cervical cancer care.[9] This twinning of care takes advantage of existing infrastructure and personnel and HIV patients' routine visits to serve those most vulnerable to cancer. During a spring 2018 visit to Malawi to assist with cervical cancer guideline development, I saw the benefits of this program taking place in a local HIV care clinic. Women would show up hours before their appointments to wait on benches, and during that time, an educator taught them about the HPV virus and cervical cancer screening. The clinic also offered rooms where patients could receive VIA screening while waiting for their HIV care – without losing their places in line! This combination of awareness-raising and testing resulted in daily VIA screening for about twenty-five women.

By conjoining services, governments amplify prevention access for all people with cervixes, but especially HIV patients six times more likely to develop cervical cancer. In the first twenty-two months of the PEPFAR program, over 1 million women (1,014,605) were screened, and 65 percent of those who needed follow-up treatment were able to receive it. Eighty-five percent of participants received their first-ever cervical cancer screening, and almost 14,000 cases of cervical cancer were suspected after those first VIA examinations.[10] Together with local governments, this global initiative hoisted large stones in the waters, breaking waves across the waters menaced by cervical cancer.

In the United States, meanwhile, parts of which continue to struggle with rising cervical cancer rates, one state has risen to the momentous challenge of disease elimination, beginning with extending screening to its hardest hit rural populations. In Alabama, a group representing the spheres of academia, citizen-volunteer organizations, and public health is collectively working toward improving cervical cancer services – including HPV vaccination, screening, follow-up, treatment, and care – with the goal of ultimately eradicating this significant "public health problem" from the entire state. Dubbed "Operation Wipe Out," this collaborative push to initially boost state screening rates has dropped its first stone in an east-central area of the state known as Chambers County, where cervical cancer incidence is almost double that of the entire state. Operation Wipe Out started in fall 2022 after months of pre-planning. Through its unique cross-section of community partnerships with such organizations as the Rotary Club, the University of Alabama at Birmingham, and TogetHER for Health, Operation Wipe Out has tailored educational materials to meet the varying needs of public health facilities across Alabama. The group's first pilot screening project, for instance, reached hundreds of Alabama women, some of whom had never before been screened. Initiatives such as these create a demand for services that were previously unavailable or hadn't yet been accessed, a demand the group hopes will build momentum toward ensuring these needs are fulfilled in future. The efforts of Operation Wipe Out represent a ripple in a great ocean of change this state hopes to become a wave.

As the world tries to "get to enough," innovations like lower-cost HPV-DNA testing and VIA testing assisted by artificial intelligence, as well as creative, collaborative partnerships in public health are tremendous ripples we want to see break into waves. But the ironic downside to such innovation is that, as more precancerous cells are found, larger numbers of people with cervixes will require care.

The Next Wave: Innovations in Treatment of Pre-Cancer

One way lower-income countries are combating the high costs of treatment for cervical cancer is by opting for lower-cost and lower-maintenance thermal ablation, which the WHO endorsed in 2019 as a safe and effective alternative to standard cryotherapy. In cryotherapy, a cooled probe freezes pre-cancerous cells; in thermal ablation, a heated probe destroys pre-cancerous cells. Thermal ablation treatment only takes a minute – as opposed to seven minutes for cryotherapy – and doesn't require the purchase and distribution of gas canisters ordinarily used for cryotherapy. Thermal ablation machines are lightweight, can be solar powered, and are easier to sterilize and clean than cryotherapy units. And a single thermal ablation unit costs about $1,500 USD. Lower-income countries like Namibia, Malawi, Kenya, and Botswana are already making use of this quicker, less expensive treatment option that will allow for more patients to be served.

But innovations like these work only when women show up for the procedures. A wonderful organization called Grounds for Health that began as a volunteer-run endeavor to bring screening to women in Oaxaca, Mexico – just a ripple – has since become an international flood. Grounds for Health understood that location and time were real barriers to access for women. The group decided to bring screening to busy and isolated women by using a "meet them where they are" approach, often working in partnership with local health care organizations and coffee cooperatives to make screening an easier, even on-the-job event. Now an internationally recognized nonprofit, with programs in Ethiopia, Kenya, Mexico, Nicaragua, Peru, and Tanzania, Grounds for Health has screened more than 100,000 women, treated several thousand women for pre-cancer, and provided clinical training for more than 400 health care providers. They have garnered major support from the coffee industry and established international partnerships with groups such as PEPFAR, Pink Ribbon Red Ribbon, and others with similar aims.

Like Teal Sisters, what began as a ripple has surged into substantial swells in the effort to eliminate cervical cancer once and for all. And this sort of work is critical to any hope of elimination: unless we reach out to marginalized women, we will never reach all women.

The Ocean Is Vast: Casting a Wider Net

Grounds for Health's particular attention to communities centered in the global supply chains for coffee, tea, cut flowers, and cocoa – working women laboring in lower-income countries – is an example of the laser focus required by every country and organization to reach previously unreachable persons with cervixes, including those marginalized by race, ethnicity, sexual orientation, income, or geographic location. Lower-income and higher-income countries alike must meet this challenge – and thankfully we've seen the first of many needed "pebbles" being tossed in those waters as well.

In the United States, thoughtful research around uptake of the cervical cancer vaccine among Indigenous peoples has accounted for differing cultural lenses and allowed HPV vaccine advocates to tailor their messages accordingly. A 2016 study found that mothers who received HPV education on the Hopi reservation in northeastern Arizona were nearly twice as likely to initiate vaccination for their daughters, compared with their less-vaccine-aware counterparts.[11] In addition, researchers found increased interest in and willingness to receive the vaccine when mother–daughter pairs were offered HPV vaccine education concurrently. This understanding that a Native American tribe's health decisions are based more on community perceptions and influence – in this case, between generations of mothers and daughters – reflects the value of culturally appropriate health initiatives. These findings offer hope for increasing vaccine uptake among people whose cervical cancer screening rates are unconscionably low in a higher-income, widely resourced country like the United States.

The ripple of this small pebble of research prompted an influential organization to pick up a large rock and see what kind of splash it would make. The American Indian Cancer Foundation designed a national, cross-generational prevention event for January 21, 2020, they called "Turquoise Tuesday." Event organizers created culturally appropriate informational materials on cervical cancer, featuring infographics specific to Indigenous populations and regional data on specific tribes to raise awareness about disease spread.[12,13] Native American women were encouraged to don native turquoise jewelry and take to social media to encourage friends and family to get Pap smears and vaccinate their children against HPV. The campaign made their online resources more culturally appropriate, directly targeting the health care providers within these communities.

The successes of the American Indian Cancer Foundation are consistent with a 2020, U.S.-based systematic review.[14] This research supported the value of population-sensitive communication for increasing vaccine uptake among minority adolescents and young adults in higher-income countries. When researchers looked at existing one-size-fits-all systems for reaching out to would-be patients – including appointment reminders and other means of improving HPV vaccine uptake – they found "limited evidence" of their benefit. Like Karen and the Teal Sisters, the American Indian Cancer Foundation was uniquely qualified to speak to and advocate for its community's needs, and the community responded in kind.

The experience of Arizona's Navajo Nation represents another example of incorporating cultural sensitivity into HPV vaccination, earning this group a national award for its efforts. The medical team for the Chinle Service Unit, which serves 35,000 people in the heart of the Navajo Nation, similarly worked with community members to combine HPV vaccination with a traditional coming-of-age ceremony, called Kinaaldá, which celebrates a girl's first period and marks the transition into adulthood. Among girls served by the unit, a whopping 82.7 percent completed their vaccination.[15] In 2018, the Association of American Cancer Institutes, in partnership with the Centers for Disease Control and Prevention and the American Cancer Society, touted the Chinle health center for its exceptionally high HPV vaccination rates – one of the most successful outcomes of all ten pediatric practices honored across the county. How fitting to weave the receipt of this life-saving vaccine into a rite of passage, thus launching girls into womanhood with ironclad protection against cervical cancer.

In another example of the use of tailored messaging, the UK-based LGBT Foundation developed a series of supportive interventions to reach lesbian and bisexual women, trans men, and nonbinary persons, groups traditionally underserved and drastically underscreened.[16] The foundation educated clinic practitioners and support staff to sensitively and respectfully engage with these patients. Their initiatives included an online training tool kit providing gender-sensitive screening invitations, sample notes for recording examinations, and other forms of information sharing that took into account this group's unique needs. Dr. Alison Berner, a British medical oncologist with a special interest in gender identity, described the work of the LGBT Foundation as a "critical intervention" on behalf of the LGBT community. Dr. Berner was a lead author for a recent statement issued by the Joint Collegiate Council for Oncology and the Association of Cancer Physicians that discussed the need to overcome the current health care barriers for those who don't identify as heterosexual. "I hope these commitments will be the start of a sea change that prioritises individual patient needs in cancer care," she said, "to provide true personalized medicine, and improve outcomes not only for LGBTQ+ patients, but all minority groups."[17]

Ripples, Waves, Tsunamis, Sea Changes: Where Does Government Fit In?

These small- and large-scale innovations demonstrate exciting ripples across the waters of cervical cancer prevention. Researchers, scientists, and manufacturers who seek more effective, less expensive, and more reliable ways to prevent, screen, and treat cervical cancer are essential to the elimination effort – as are local, community-imbedded stakeholders like the Teal Sisters and the American Indian Cancer Foundation. When these powerful advocates work together with weighty, government-backed organizations like the United Kingdom's National Health Service or the Zambian Health Ministry, they create more of a splash than a ripple. And behemoth agencies such as USAID, the Global Fund, PEPFAR, Gavi, and Unitaid that commit to supporting the WHO's cervical cancer elimination strategy with funding for things like training and equipment for lower-income countries whip up waves to great effect.

But the fight against cervical cancer needs more than waves. It needs storms of political will. It needs a tsunami of political passion. It needs a sea change.

With health budgets, ministry staffing, and political clout, governments are uniquely positioned to bring about this change. While grassroots efforts are highly effective and necessary, when a national government puts its considerable and sustained clout behind a health care initiative, success gets a substantial boost.

The Canadian government has generally been willing to put money and policy behind equitably decreasing the country's cervical cancer rates, possibly owing to its historical provision of universal public health care. In recent years, the country's health care ministry has focused on improving vaccination and cervical cancer screening rates for marginalized First Nations, Inuit, and Metis women. The Canadian Partnership Against Cancer has also been working nationwide with public health agencies, cancer agencies, and academic researchers to meet the country's 2019 to 2029 Canadian Strategy for Cancer Control, and in February 2020, hosted an Elimination of Cervical Cancer Summit calling for the end of cervical cancer in Canada by 2040.[18] Both the health ministry strategy and the cancer agency summit paid special attention to the needs of First Nations, Inuit, and Metis women who develop cervical cancer at rates threefold higher than do non-Indigenous Canadian women, and die at rates fourfold higher than their non-Indigenous counterparts.[19]

New Zealand is another higher-income country willing to support traditionally marginalized groups by extending cervical cancer prevention outside the mainstream. In 2020, the country developed a national media outreach plan to screen more twenty- to twenty-five-year-old New Zealand women, focusing in particular on those with Maori and Pacific ethnicities. The "Give Your Cervix Some Screen Time" campaign offers another example of targeting an underscreened population.[20]

In the United States, it has taken time to see the government involved in thoughtful, culturally sensitive messaging, but these efforts are yielding results, with citizens showing an increased willingness to consider HPV vaccination. When the vaccine was first launched in 2006, government messaging touted its power to prevent sexually transmitted infection. And indeed, that's what vaccination does: stop HPV transmission in its tracks. But this messaging backfired by heightening parents' fears about the vaccine encouraging female promiscuity, resulting in only 19 percent of eligible teens getting vaccinated during the launch. As a result, U.S. medical societies – representing oncologists, pediatricians, obstetricians, gynecologists, and family medical providers – have since diverted the emphasis toward the vaccine's lifesaving, cancer-stopping powers, and media campaigns from state and local health departments, along with the Centers for Disease Control and Prevention (CDC), are using a similar, health-focused message to promote HPV vaccination.[21] By drawing the public's attention away from sexual transmission and toward inoculating girls against cancer, public perceptions toward the HPV vaccine have begun to shift – a phenomenon I've noticed among patients in my medical practice.

The lesson? Public health messaging is a powerful tool, but it must be wielded with great care. In 2021, 77 percent of U.S. adolescents had received one HPV vaccination dose and 62 percent had received the full recommended series.[22] While the United States remains far below its cervical cancer–protecting potential, the HPV vaccine has come a long way in this country with the help of a much-needed shift in attitudes.

A Global Model of Vision, Tenacity – and Taking the Long View

Cervical cancer prevention initiatives on the part of governments in New Zealand, the United Kingdom, the United States, and Canada demonstrate just a few heartening examples of higher-income countries employing national assets to spare the lives of often-overlooked citizens. But Australia offers the gold standard. In terms of the world's richest countries, no country has shown more determination and commitment to ending cervical cancer than this one. Australia, a relatively isolated "island unto itself," has channeled considerable resources into preventing cervical cancer, and by 2035 is on track to being the first country to eliminate the disease.[23,24] Australia's global leadership serves as an inspiration to other countries, showing how to free women from the terrible toll of cervical cancer through its use of policy changes, improved access to prevention and treatment, advocacy and communication campaigns, and attention to underresourced population groups.

How did Australia get there? With tenacity and vision, and a willingness to take the long view: a slow, steady approach.[25] Australia introduced its national cervical cancer screening program in 1991. In a country that provides subsidized medical care, this meant that virtually all Australian women had access to screening. And yet the Royal College of Pathologists of Australasia[26] attributes much of the program's success not only to provision of "free" services, but also to the national coordination effort. The Australian government set up "Pap test registers" in each state and territory to ensure women were taking part in regular screening. These disparate registries morphed into a more efficient federal database, creating a "failsafe mechanism for following-up women with abnormalities," a monitoring system for Pap smear quality control, and a standardized patient management system. The government could identify regions with low screening rates and generate the political will and funding to boost these programs accordingly.

In 2006, the Australian Therapeutic Goods Administration approved the HPV vaccine for use. The national government had already developed systems for distributing and monitoring use of the vaccine, negotiating affordable rates with suppliers, and covering the procurement cost. To maximize vaccination rates over the shortest period, in 2007, Australian girls twelve to eighteen began receiving the vaccine at school, while Australian women eighteen to twenty-six were vaccinated in physicians' offices. The expansion of the vaccine's eligible age range – and the government's willingness to pay for it – drastically diminished HPV-cancer spread. In the first two years of introduction, 80 percent of Australian school-aged girls and 50 percent of young women eighteen to twenty-six got vaccinated, making the country the world's first in establishing a national HPV program and vaccinating the majority of its target population. After the program's first three years, Australia was in a position to scale back and switch focus toward school-based vaccination of girls twelve to fourteen – now a standard feature of the country's HPV vaccination program.

As part of that program, the Australian government funded a national vaccine registry to track participation rates – valuable data in garnering ongoing support and helpful feedback for improving its cervical cancer prevention efforts. Wisely, the country's federal health ministry linked its Pap smear registry with the new vaccine registry, creating a powerful means to track how, when, and why women were using and benefiting from HPV vaccination and screening. This system allowed a rapid response to areas of the program that needed strengthening or changing to take advantage of all opportunities to prevent cervical cancer. These are just some of the measures Australia took to demonstrate their commitment to saving lives through cervical cancer prevention – requiring an enviable level of foresight and political will – while demonstrating that this cancer can be eliminated.

In September 2020, I asked Dr. Suzanne Garland, an Australian and global leader in HPV vaccine research, to explain what sparked the country's exceptional participation in HPV vaccination. "Public health is valued here," she said. "What's more, the vaccine was offered for free, and made widely available in schools and in clinics across the country." Dr. Garland noted that Australia's introduction to the HPV vaccine benefited from Dr. Ian Fraser – one of the HPV vaccine developers – being named "Australian of the Year" in 2006. Dr. Fraser used his celebrity status to promote the vaccine. Similarly, Janette Howard, wife of then-Australian prime minister John Howard, kept the prospect of disease front and center by revealing in October 2006 that she'd been treated for cervical cancer a decade earlier. "All of these factors helped the whole country to know about the vaccine, and encouraged its uptake," Dr. Garland said. When a well-known person is willing to be up front and personal about the disease, much as the Teal Sisters' Karen Nakawala discovered in Zambia, it allows the public to be more comfortable with taking part in prevention measures.

It did not take long for Australia to see a return on its HPV vaccination investment. Within a year of initiating the nationwide program, an important piece of evidence emerged. Researchers tracking available data learned that the genital wart rate in heterosexual males had decreased by 50 percent – a key marker revealing lower circulation of the HPV virus. In just one year, a major source of cancer had begun to disappear.

I distinctly remember hearing those astonishing Australian results in 2010 at one of the largest scientific meetings around HPV disease, the twenty-sixth annual International Papillomavirus Meeting in Montreal, Quebec. This study was the first to establish the possibility of herd immunity against genital warts via use of the HPV vaccine, indicating that lowered disease rates among vaccinated people would grant protection to the unvaccinated.[27] These results promised a direct benefit for the fight against cervical cancer. They allowed the outside world to witness proof of the HPV vaccine's effectiveness.

As a result of many years of early and consistent vaccine use, and in addition to experiencing the vaccine's direct cancer-fighting benefits, Australia is enjoying a significant drop in abnormal Pap smears. These results have underlined the advantage of combining two highly effective methods of prevention against the disease.

And yet, in spite of Australia's outstanding successes against cervical cancer, the country remains beleaguered by inequitable participation in health care, an issue facing all higher-income countries. Australia's cervical cancer prevention program was designed to be far reaching and accessible, but some communities have yet to see the benefits of publicly funded screening and vaccination. Aboriginal women, in particular, have traditionally demonstrated lower screening rates and thereby suffer higher rates of cervical cancer than their non-Aboriginal counterparts. According to a Cancer Institute of New South Wales report, Aboriginal females are 2.5 times more likely to develop cervical cancer. Moreover, they are 3.8 times as likely to die of the disease; only 56 percent are likely to survive cervical cancer five years after diagnosis, compared with 72 percent of other Australian females.[28]

One of the distinct differences between Australia and other higher-income countries, however, is the government's apparent understanding that as long as marginalized populations and regions remain underserved, the country cannot meet its goal of cervical cancer elimination. In response, a variety of Australian governmental and nongovernmental organizations are working together to address notable internal disparities in cervical cancer rates. The Cancer Institute NSW launched a culturally specific cervical cancer education program for Aboriginal women known as the "NSW Aboriginal Cervical Screening Network." This network offers opportunities for Aboriginal health care providers to share resources and insights with those who work in non-Aboriginal health care environments and with Aboriginal community representatives. Its purpose is to foster non-Aboriginal understanding and appreciation of the distinct health care needs of Aboriginals. These network-sponsored opportunities include training workshops across the state of New South Wales for women from local NSW health districts, primary health networks, and Aboriginal medical services to address the lifesaving importance of cervical cancer screening, and HPV vaccination as the key to prevention. In September 2019, an inaugural NSW Aboriginal Cervical Screening Forum purposefully addressed lower cervical cancer screening rates among the country's Indigenous women, the ongoing goal of a government determined to see the disease swept away within its borders.

In Australia – just as in Zambia through the work of the Teal Sisters – the government has included a partnership with women in its vision, investing significant resources to elevate their voices and share their wisdom directly with those most affected. This sort of partnership is emblematic of a government's commitment to universal – and equitable – cervical cancer care for all.

Zambia: A Lower-Income Country's Commitment

Australia's determination to offer vaccination, screening, and treatment to all offers an inspirational example, one many lower-income countries would like to follow. Among them,

Zambia is making sizable strides, having achieved the herculean task of developing a permanent, government-run, and government-funded cervical cancer screening program. What started as a donor-funded research program to use VIA for cervical cancer screening has since evolved into a long-standing, national health ministry–supported venture. The health ministry has extended its investment by creating a supervisory position to oversee the program, allowing ongoing training and supervision for VIA providers and the expansion of sites and clinics offering VIA. The person in charge of this program was Dr. Sharon Kampabwe.

Speaking to me over Zoom in the winter of 2021, Dr. Kampabwe weighed in on her government's success in making cervical cancer prevention and treatment a health care priority, in the hopes of other countries applying similar oversight. In Zambia, nurses represent the cervical cancer screening-and-treatment workforce, and patients with pre-cancer are referred to physicians only when they need loop electrosurgical excision procedure (LEEP) treatment over and above thermal ablation or cryotherapy – or if cancer is already present. Zambian nurses run their own supervision and quality improvement programs and have greater opportunities to establish patient rapport. The country's willingness to allow midwives or nurses to serve in addition to physicians deepens the ranks of health care providers. Dr. Kampabwe attributed program gains in VIA screening to the country's ability to train and retain health care providers by encouraging greater involvement of its female workforce and expanding the notion of what constitutes a qualified provider.

What made Zambia unique, Dr. Kampabwe said, was its choice to fund an ongoing cervical cancer screening program even before the WHO announced its global call for cervical cancer elimination. After publicly committing to the WHO strategy, other lower-income countries can look to Zambia as an example of a country's willingness to tackle its own obstacles to cervical cancer prevention without waiting for the world's permission.

In this context, you can see how Karen and the Teal Sisters grew their powerful advocacy role exponentially. But it's important to note that the Teal Sisters were only able to do so alongside a preexisting cervical cancer screening system. The absence of such an infrastructure remains a persistent, pernicious problem in attempting to agitate the placid waters: the world's common mindset of "cervical cancer forever." Unless one ripple – say, a survivor willing to tell her story – is met by another ripple – other people who meet that story with support and enthusiasm and invitation – and another ripple – the actual access people with cervixes need – then the waters fall still, again and again.

Churning the Waters toward a "Sea Change"

Australia's and Zambia's perseverance in offering nationwide cervical cancer care reminds us that steadiness and persistence can lead to change, despite the monumental tide against it. And, as I write these words, the scourge of cervical cancer happens to be in the spotlight: the WHO's call for global elimination has brought the disease front and center. The subsequent attention and availability of donor funds and donor resources – in combination with new and promising screening technologies and grassroots awareness raising and advocacy – reflect hopeful ripples in stopping this deadly disease. International and national organizations, along with deeply caring and dedicated individuals, are driving global and domestic initiatives to vastly improve women's chances of surviving cervical cancer. The battle has begun. From pebble-tossers to boulder-launchers, we'll require an ocean-sized swell of support.

The global call for cervical cancer elimination asks that by the year 2030, all countries achieve 90 percent HPV vaccine coverage, 70 percent screening coverage, and 90 percent access to treatment for cervical pre-cancer and cancer, including access to palliative care – aspirational goals, for sure. All 194 member countries of the United Nations have agreed to these targets that, if met, would save 300,000 lives by 2030.[29,30] But all of the efforts we've visited in this chapter are not enough – have demonstrably not been enough – to address the annual and rising number of global cervical cancer deaths.

Every ripple of hope we've explored in this chapter relies on multiple factors to become a wave. A one-dose HPV vaccine option only works when countries have access to and can afford that one dose. Thermal ablation is only an option when countries can afford the necessary tools and trained providers to offer the treatment. People with cervixes can only enjoy the precision and confidence of an HPV-DNA test if they have access to it and can afford it. Survivors and their allies can only advocate for things that communities and governments are willing to budget for, fund, procure, and provide. All the nonprofits and donors in the world cannot overcome scarcity of infrastructure, personnel, tests, equipment, and money without government-level political passion and will.

And all of this needs to happen in every single country.

These efforts are going to require a sea change in how we value women, a profound transformation in political will around women's health and their value to society – the health of all women, the value of all women, regardless of race, orientation, ethnicity, income, or geography. Only when a country's government and ministries of health and finance decide that women are worth their time, money, and energy can this killer cancer receive the attention and funding it deserves. Only when we see all women around the world with equal value will we turn the tide on cervical cancer.

When will the value and worth of women to their families, their villages, their communities, and their countries be enough? When will the care and wisdom they offer all of us be enough? When will the world have had enough of a cancer preventable on the basis of where you live? Change has begun with tiny circles created by small pebbles; we've seen stones and a few boulders, waves and storms.

I want a sea change. No, more than that: I want a tsunami.

In the race to stop the spread of this virulent cancer, change cannot come soon enough.

15 WANTED: MEN TO CHAMPION THE MOVEMENT

The rising chorus for change in this book rings truest for those born with female reproductive systems. As it should. After all, cervical cancer strikes persons with cervixes. But it would make little sense to exclude men while expecting one half of the population to wage this battle by itself. Besides asking men to play a role in diminishing deadly HPV spread, they can contribute to and support the cause in unique and innumerable ways. To do otherwise would be shortsighted, even foolish. Men benefit greatly from keeping women alive.

Let's take a closer look at what men can do to protect, and even covet, their best interests. How can persons without cervixes champion the cervical cancer cause?

The answer to that question is that men can do a great deal. Their connection to cervical cancer, in fact, goes right back to the origins of the disease. From a purely biological perspective, men – often unwittingly – contribute to the incidence of cervical cancer when they transmit HPV during sex. It stands to reason, then, that men own their part in HPV transmission and show initiative in breaking that transmission chain.

Men can be proactive in countless other ways as well. They can play a critical role in supporting and advocating for those who may acquire cervical cancer; every woman is some man's sister, wife, partner, friend, or mother. Men can bring about profound progress in disease prevention by working to transform patriarchal norms and laws. And they can support women in leadership positions and empower them to make their own health care decisions. These efforts are instrumental toward the larger goal of reducing cervical cancer rates.

What's more, simply by stepping up on behalf of a person with a cervix, a man broadcasts a message about women's importance, reflecting just how valuable they are to his own health and well-being, how instrumental they are to his larger community. His actions are transmuted into something that's both life affirming and life giving. As every woman who's ever struggled with cervical cancer has learned: we need both men and women to support and sustain us – we can't do this journey alone.

The Power of a Supportive Partner

"Keeping women alive" is at its most personal when men are supporting a loved one suffering from cervical cancer. A man's role in a private battle with cervical cancer is to be a steady, supportive ally. Supporters are vital to every cancer journey. Not all women suffering from cervical cancer have or choose a male to be their champion. Fortunately, support comes in all shapes and sizes, genders, and compositions, and that includes support groups. But any man informed by compassion and sensitivity can make a vital difference in improving the personal toll of cervical cancer.

Loretta, a resident of La Habra, California, relied heavily on the support of her male partner during her battle with cervical cancer. Loretta was forty-eight and had been married to Jeff for eleven years when she received her devastating diagnosis in 2014. Although her previous Pap smears had tested normal, Loretta learned she had cervical cancer while being treated for abnormal bleeding and what appeared to be a non-cancerous fibroid. Both she and her gynecologist had assumed cancer wasn't a consideration, and were shocked when her biopsy results showed "aggressive cervical cancer." When Jeff heard the news, "he put his head in his hands, put his head down, and just cried. He was devastated."

Despite the upheaval accompanying Loretta's diagnosis, she was grateful for her husband's unwavering support. "Jeff sprang into action for me." As U.S. residents, Jeff and Loretta were lucky to have private insurance and access to a higher-income country's medical care system. However, Loretta's insurance plan lacked coverage for a crucial leader of her future care team. Its approved list of providers didn't include a gynecologic oncologist, someone with the necessary training and experience to direct her treatment plan. As she struggled to cope with her diagnosis, she needed to mount the energy to advocate that her insurance company add gynecologic oncologists to its list. "This was where Jeff took over," Loretta said. "He made phone calls, figured out the systems, and kept track of everything so that I could go see a gynecologic oncologist for my cancer surgery. It was so much work and took a great deal of time. I cannot imagine having to deal with that at the same time I was adjusting to needing cancer treatment."

An MRI scan prior to treatment ramped up pressures for the couple, revealing that Loretta's cervical tumor had grown from the size of a quarter to that of a lemon – agonizingly close to the maximum size surgery could remove. "We had to move fast," Loretta said. "Fortunately, with all of Jeff's phone calls and help with the paperwork, we got a gynecologic oncologist in our network, and I was able to have my surgical treatment for my cancer – a radical hysterectomy and removal of my lymph nodes – quite quickly."

From Supportive Partner to Advocate

While surgery confirmed confinement of the cancer to Loretta's uterus, she'd required four blood transfusions and faced an arduous recovery. "Of course, Jeff was so helpful in that time," she said. She needed Jeff's emotional support as she wrestled with the knowledge that her cancer could have been prevented if she'd been born years later when the HPV vaccine was available. "My tumor was adenocarcinoma caused by HPV-18," she said. "It broke my heart that there were no HPV vaccine shots for my age that could have prevented me from getting this cancer."

After Loretta recovered some of her strength, she felt compelled to help other women by spreading the word about HPV, the HPV vaccine, and the dangers of cervical cancer (Figure 15.1). She established Teal Ladies Move Mountains (www.tealladiesmove mountains.com) to raise awareness about gynecologic cancers, and began speaking and giving interviews about her experiences with cervical cancer. But it was not just Loretta who moved into advocacy. Jeff was equally driven to make a difference.

During Loretta's illness, and in the years thereafter, Jeff moved beyond the role of supportive partner to actively raising awareness about the disease. As a La Habra policeman, Jeff and his fellow officers capitalized on January's "cervical cancer month" to create their own campaign. In January 2015, and again in 2016, they produced magnets in the shape of teal-colored ribbons – the symbolic color of cervical cancer prevention – and endeavored to raise awareness by displaying them on detachment police cars. Their efforts garnered extensive local media coverage and prompted calls of support from women as far away as Cincinnati, Ohio. Loretta's husband and his fellow officers reflect just one way men can support loved ones directly and indirectly, by attracting public attention toward cervical cancer prevention.

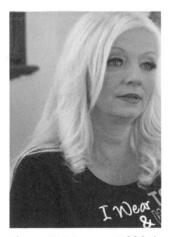

Figure 15.1 Loretta Goldthrite-Goldthwaite, a Cervical cancer survivor.

Breaking the Transmission Chain

Men like Jeff are instrumental to the battle against cervical cancer. But through the spread of cancer-causing HPV, they also represent one-half of its transmission chain. While persons with cervixes can acquire HPV from males or females – including those born with female reproductive organs who don't identify as female – most women acquire it from having sex with males. HPV spreads quickly and easily. By the time a woman has had three or more sexual partners, more than 50 percent of the time she'll have been infected with HPV. More than 80 percent of adults acquire an HPV infection during their lifetimes. Yet few men, or women, are attuned to the risks of HPV every time they have sex.

Fortunately, most HPV infections will clear, and most will not feature the high-risk, cancer-causing types of HPV, such as the HPV-18 type that Loretta had. But as Loretta and Jeff discovered the hard way, HPV can develop into cervical cancer and seemingly go on to strike healthy women at random – often in the prime of their lives. Men are in a key position to abate this deadly transfer. A male partner's willingness to use condoms is still one of the best and most straightforward ways men can diminish HPV spread. Condom use can prevent more than 60 percent of male-to-female HPV transmission and provide near-total prevention of HIV transmission and pregnancy. But because condoms cover the shaft of the penis and not the surrounding skin, and because HPV transfer can occur from skin-to-skin sexual contact outside of the condom's protective covering, condom use does not eliminate all HPV transmission.

Another way males can decrease HPV transmission to females is through penile circumcision. In addition to protecting against HPV, male circumcision – whether it takes place at birth or in adulthood – can prevent sexually transmitted infections from being passed on to female partners. Circumcision protects against both HPV and HIV infections. However, while the World Health Organization recommends male circumcision to lower HIV transmission rates, and many countries and cultures encourage this practice, using male circumcision to decrease HPV – and hence, cervical cancer – remains relatively unfamiliar and is rarely discussed.

A 2020 Australian study used computer modeling to evaluate the effects of voluntary medical male circumcision on cervical cancer in Tanzania – a country with a high burden of HIV disease and cervical cancer.[1] The authors predicted that male circumcision in Tanzania would have prevented nearly 3,000 cervical cancer cases and more than 1,000 cervical cancer deaths between 1995 and 2020. The authors also predicted that by 2070, voluntary male circumcision would have lowered Tanzanian cervical cancer incidence and mortality rates by 28 percent. The Tanzanian study reflects similar findings from a 2017 U.S.-based systematic review of circumcised males and their female partners. Researchers looked at global findings from nine cervical cancer studies and five studies on cervical pre-cancer. They found that male circumcision helped to protect female partners from developing both cervical cancer and pre-cancer.[2] And yet, despite the proven efficacy of male circumcision in preventing cervical cancer, this practice has failed to garner widespread discussion, media interest, or consideration as a public health policy. Given the divided personal opinions about male circumcision, and the lack of precedent for using an intervention on males to prevent a "female disease," it's not surprising that the practice has yet to be incorporated into the field of women's health – regardless of its capacity for reducing disease spread.

The Complications of Male HPV Vaccination

While encouraging males to use condoms or get circumcised immediately lowers HPV transmission, and thereby cervical cancer, HPV vaccination for boys circumvents the virus by preventing males from being infected with the most common cancer-causing types of HPV in the first place. As with any inoculation against an infectious virus, the HPV vaccine protects the vaccinated person as well as the people that person comes into contact with. A boy who is vaccinated against future HPV infection protects his future partners too.

When, in 2011, the United States first recommended the HPV vaccine for use in males twelve to twenty-one, I remember telling my boys, then aged fifteen and seventeen, "I do not want you to ever give a sexual partner the virus that can cause cervical cancer. Of course, the vaccine protects you, but it also allows you to protect future partners." Their pediatrician said I was one of the first parents to request male vaccination. As the mother of sons and a physician intimately acquainted with the devastation of cervical cancer, I readily saw the advantage of protecting my sons and their future partners from HPV-related cancers.

But in 2011, the world wasn't battling a shortage of the HPV vaccine. International aid organizations had yet to commit to funding HPV vaccine purchase for lower-income countries, and so global demand could meet supply. So when the CDC Advisory Committee on Immunization Practices voted, in October 2011, to recommend HPV vaccination for twelve- to twenty-one-year-old U.S. boys, it could clearly justify that recommendation, especially since female uptake of the vaccination had been slow and stalled at just 30 percent.[3] In addition to arguing that male vaccination prevented the spread of HPV to females, the CDC's vote took into account the direct benefits of preventing HPV-associated cancers in males – head, neck, penile, and anal cancers – even while acknowledging that male cancers were less common than cervical cancer.

But when the CDC debated vaccinating males, health economists agreed (and still do) that vaccinating females against HPV remains a better investment, because HPV poses the greater cancer risk for females (Figure 15.2). The WHO has consistently supported giving girls first priority for the vaccine, in keeping with their initial 2009 recommendation that girls nine to fourteen seek HPV vaccination. When more countries found funding for the vaccine, global supply could not keep pace with demand, and that meant not enough shots to go around for all females and males wanting the vaccine. As a result, WHO

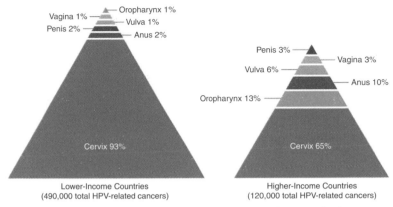

Figure 15.2 Comparison of cervical cancer with incidence of other HPV cancers Reproduced from BMJ, Rahangdale, L., Mungo, C., O'Connor, S., Chibwesha, C.J., Brewer, N.T., 379:e070115, 2022 with permission from BMJ Publishing Group Ltd.

vaccination recommendations have remained largely – and justifiably – female-focused.

Amid a global HPV vaccine shortage – ongoing as of 2022 – the WHO has reiterated its girls-first focus. The WHO's vaccination advisory board, SAGE, called for a halt of male vaccination as of 2019 until supply levels improve.[4] For girls in lower-income countries with rare to nonexistent annual screening or treatment services, the vaccine can be their one-and-only option for preventing cervical cancer long-term. SAGE's recommendations to temporary halt male vaccination, under the auspices of the WHO, are just that – recommendations. They're not binding. Hence, 44 percent of all higher-income countries, including England, Australia, and the United States, currently offer male HPV vaccination.[5]

In trying to eliminate cervical cancer, using a limited HPV vaccine supply to protect males in countries with the highest cervical-cancer burden becomes particularly problematic. A decade before the HPV vaccine fell prey to a global shortage – when the WHO suggested male vaccination for countries whose young girls had achieved high coverage – countries with sufficient public health funds began vaccinating young men. And while most lower-income countries have yet to recommend routine male HPV vaccination, their typically patriarchal foundations make them vulnerable to practices favoring males, such as male vaccination – decisions that further diminish the supply for females. The inherent problem of cultures prizing boys over girls is one of the reasons to strive for higher vaccination rates in females before considering vaccination for males. These societal pressures take the conversation away from stopping cervical cancer.

It would be ideal to offer the HPV vaccine to everyone. But the current policy of vaccinating boys in higher-income countries dangerously depletes the supply of this precious resource in countries vastly more vulnerable to cervical cancer. Until supply increases, hard decisions must be made. The HPV vaccine is a finite resource. Every time the HPV vaccine is diverted for use in males, one fewer dose is available for females in the precarious global supply chain. It is my hope that both men and women in the position to make decisions around access to the HPV vaccine pay close attention to women's greater vulnerability to cancers caused by HPV.

The HPV vaccine is a finite resource. Every time the HPV vaccine is diverted for use in males, one fewer dose is available for females in the precarious global supply chain.

Dismantling the Patriarchy

Persons with cervixes are best served when society bands together to address what gets in the way of equal access to cervical cancer care. Alongside women, men can advocate for disease prevention services as a form of health care for all. Specifically, men can demand, on behalf of women, a more equitable distribution of resources toward prevention and early treatment of this disease. Men have a unique role when it comes to dismantling the more insidious barriers to women's health care. If we think about patriarchy being a system – be it institutional or informal – in which men hold the power and women are largely excluded from it, then men are ideally positioned to chip away at those barriers, to turn the sledgehammer and the paper cutter of patriarchy on itself and free women and men alike.

To meet these goals, men will need to acknowledge and address outdated or misguided beliefs about women's bodies, about women's role in society, and about women's autonomy in accessing care and making choices about it. Men must support women in leadership – publicly and privately – and empower them as they advocate for their own health and global health overall.

These changes will take time. Convincing men in male-dominated cultures to encourage and support cervical cancer screening for their women and champion cervical cancer elimination means challenging deep-rooted beliefs: beliefs that the female's genital region belongs to her male partner and is only for him to see or govern; beliefs that women's bodies are dangerous or dirty; beliefs that disease should be the source of women's shame. Within the confines of these beliefs, men may discourage or even forbid their wives from receiving the pelvic examinations necessary for cervical cancer screening. They may shame and blame their partners, rather than supporting them in their suffering. Addressing these practices – and the complex belief systems underlying them – requires respectful enlightenment, and tangible, practical ways to help men exit the prison of patriarchy that binds both sexes. These challenges are not confined to institutionally patriarchal countries. As I've said before, patriarchy seeps in everywhere. Upending these structures means that men everywhere must dig out and confront the wrong-headed internal messages that prevent them from wholly supporting and advocating for women's health.

Men who draw on the support of other men become a potent force in the fight against cervical cancer. By engaging in peer-to-peer communication – men talking to men – the world's males can find consensus around women's health issues in ways that directly benefit men. Already, the direct involvement of men in HIV education and prevention has rapidly advanced research in HIV-related AIDS management and HIV death-rate reduction. There's no reason such a concerted effort can't be applied to a "woman's disease" like cervical cancer, especially in light of HIV's accelerant effect on HPV.

Teal Sisters' Karen Nakawala strongly supports male participation in the cervical cancer fight. "My husband is a big part of Teal Sisters, and he advocates his fellow men to encourage them to get their partners screened, tested, and their young girls vaccinated," she said. "We see couples come together, especially when we offer prostate screening as well. We have discovered that this is the 'winning formula' in Zambia."

"My husband is a big part of Teal Sisters, and he advocates his fellow men to encourage them to get their partners screened, tested, and their young girls vaccinated."

What's more, using male peer-to-peer education can be especially useful for reducing cervical cancer rates in cultures where men still hold power over women's health choices. When a man understands the value of cervical cancer vaccination, screening, and treatment to a woman's life and thereby his own, he is more likely to support it. When men are introduced to their own capacity for keeping women alive, they, too, can witness the power of an individual to effect change.

In addition to raising awareness of the toll of cervical cancer, men can also rely on their personal and professional power – and even occasionally cede that power – to ensure women the easiest possible access to cervical cancer screening and treatment. I witnessed an example of this form of advocacy in 2017 while working with the Namibian Ministry of Health on the country's cervical cancer screening guidelines. At that time, the ministry faced ongoing challenges in finding and training appropriate providers to perform VIA exams for cervical cancer screening and pre-cancer treatment. Clinics across Namibia had been relying primarily on male doctors and clinical officers to offer these services, because nurses, most of them female, were not authorized to place speculums in patients' vaginas or perform pelvic exams. Although this problem might seem easily remedied, the sanctioning of a well-developed training and credentialing program for nurses to perform VIA screenings did in fact require considerable persuasion and, frankly, paperwork on the part of the health ministry. In turn, Namibian women immediately gained access to this critical aspect of cervical cancer prevention, thanks to the mostly male leaders of this initiative, who willingly used and relinquished their power to accomplish this task.

Namibia's willingness to rethink health care provision for the benefit of female patients and providers marks a small but important step forward. The gargantuan, global effort to eliminate cervical cancer will require just such a mindful, steady spotlight on women. It's in men's best interest, after all, to keep women at the forefront. Men can take personal responsibility for preventing HPV transmission. They can advocate broadly for women's health, raising and echoing their voices in health care legislation and policy. And they can confront beliefs that diminish women's autonomy in health care. The quest to eliminate this preventable cancer, in fact, cannot succeed without the unwavering support, understanding, and commitment of the world's other half.

The quest to eliminate this preventable cancer, in fact, cannot succeed without the unwavering support, understanding, and commitment of the world's other half.

---

16 JOIN THE COLLECTIVE CRY OF "ENOUGH!"

It's probably clear by now that the energy, resources, and commitment needed to rid the globe of cervical cancer are vast, even daunting. As a reader, you might be asking what you can possibly do to influence this herculean effort. Isn't that for people with money to spare? Sophisticated political connections? A working knowledge of global policy decisions? As one lone human caught up in an epic, worldwide battle – does what you do matter? Can you really make a difference?

The answer, of course, is yes. You're already making a difference. You picked up a book and decided that by reading it, you could educate yourself about a cancer that continues to be a well-kept secret. Just by doing that, you can talk to people about cervical cancer and knowledgeably answer their questions, even without formal medical training. If everyone who picked up this book decided that in addition to learning and sharing more about cervical cancer, they would work toward ending it, we would see the needle shift toward fewer diagnoses and deaths.

If everyone who picked up this book decided that in addition to learning and sharing more about cervical cancer, they would work toward ending it, we would see the needle shift toward fewer diagnoses and deaths.

These efforts don't just involve money. Raising awareness of the disease and elevating its importance on a country or community's health agenda can have immediate, far-reaching effects.

Start Small, Follow Your Passion

Donations to a cause are always a start, and certainly necessary. But doing away with cervical cancer requires so much more than cash donations. Where you direct your energies is entirely up to you. When you focus on the plight of women nearby, far away, or both, you help save lives. How you choose to help may depend on where you can offer the most benefit. I would encourage you to peruse the profiles of cervical cancer support groups, prevention agencies, and other health initiatives listed in the Reader Resources section at the back of this book. Find the groups or causes you feel most comfortable with and passionate about supporting. However you choose to help marks a step toward eradicating this terrible cancer.

When the goal seems daunting, anchor it in the experiences of people who have been there. Maybe one of the people featured in this book inspired you. Follow that feeling! So many women in the journey of writing this book have inspired me, but the first woman who showed me what the word *advocacy* means and made me eager to roll up my sleeves is the founder of a cervical cancer support and prevention advocacy group called Cervivor, a woman named Tamika Felder.

The Woman Who Sparked My Desire for Change

I first met Tamika in December 2015 (Figure 16.1). We were both attending a meeting to develop HPV vaccine guidelines for the American Society of Clinical Oncology. Tamika, who lives in Baltimore, Maryland, had been invited as a former cervical cancer patient and survivor-advocate, and I was there as an HPV vaccine expert. I was inspired by Tamika's passion to change cervical cancer policy. Her desire to put survivors' stories like her own at the forefront made intuitive sense. When she and I had dinner together after that meeting, we talked about our shared passion for helping women with cervical cancer. Tamika's warm, open, and compelling spirit drew me in. Looking back, I wonder if Tamika planted the seed for this

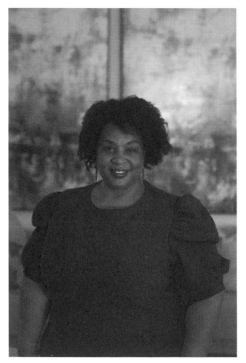

Figure 16.1 Tamika Felder, founder and chief visionary for Cervivor. Photo credit: Elyse Cosgrove Torch Pictures.

book: an idea that would eventually prompt me to nurture her vision of the transformative power of women's stories.

What Gives Me Pause: A Woman So Young with Cancer

I caught up with Tamika on Zoom five years after our first meeting. The computer screen couldn't cloak her passion – or her grief – as she waded into her personal journey with cervical cancer from such an early age. Tamika was twenty-five when she learned she had cervical cancer. Twenty-five! Tamika had been going for regular Pap smears with her childhood doctor starting at eighteen, until a negative experience with a different doctor a few years later wreaked havoc with her regimen.

When Tamika moved to Washington, D.C., for her first job in television production, she walked in to see her new doctor and was subjected to toxic and damaging remarks: "Did you know that if you were pregnant," the doctor said, "you wouldn't even know you were because of how overweight you are."

"I left without being screened for cervical cancer," Tamika said. "I just couldn't let that person do a Pap smear after those comments."

Roughly two years later, Tamika saw a different doctor for a minor skin problem, and was reminded she was overdue for cervical screening. She came back two weeks later for a Pap smear. "I remember showing up in my power suit: new professional, new job, steady income, feeling confident. Then, once I heard my results – 'carcinoma-in-situ' – I had a full-on panic attack. I had to go lie down, just to get a hold of myself."

As she recalled her shock over the results, I watched Tamika take a slow, deep breath. The anguish on her face told me she'd been pulled back to this moment. "The next day, they got me in to see the gynecology specialist who could do a colposcopy and biopsies. I remember the nurse holding my hand, because I was a wreck: emotionally, spiritually, physically. I heard the sound as they pinched my cervix for the biopsies. The nurse was trying to comfort me, but she had that look on her face that just let me know, 'This is not going to be good.'"

After confirming her cancer diagnosis, Tamika learned she needed to have a radical hysterectomy. Because of how hard this news was, her doctor encouraged Tamika to get a second opinion. "So, I saw ten doctors to get ten opinions. I saw a doctor at Harvard who told me that my cervix looked like chewed-up meat. I saw another doctor that said – since I was so young – I should be tested for HIV. I'm twenty-five. I want to have babies," she recalled. "Can you imagine just how awful that was? I couldn't even believe I had cancer. Now I was hearing I would never have children. But then also being told I should get tested for HIV – well, that was the moment the stigma of cervical cancer hit me. After that, I didn't want to tell anyone about the cervical cancer."

"I'm twenty-five. I want to have babies," she recalled. *"Can you imagine just how awful that was? I couldn't even believe I had cancer. Now I was hearing I would never have children. But then also being told I should get tested for HIV – well, that was the moment the stigma of cervical cancer hit me. After that, I didn't want to tell anyone about the cervical cancer."*

Cervical Cancer Invades Body, Mind, and Soul

In my thirty years as a practitioner, I've never heard of a patient seeking ten second opinions (let alone a patient who's been told her cervix looked like "chewed-up meat"). I asked Tamika what it took to keep going – to seek all of that additional input. "I had a lot of friends who moved mountains for me," she said. "I was looking for one doctor to say, 'All those other doctors had it wrong; you don't need a hysterectomy.' I kept asking myself, 'How is it possible I have cancer?'"

After each doctor confirmed her cancer, Tamika went ahead with the radical hysterectomy. In addition to a "terrible" post-surgical recovery and side effects from chemotherapy and radiation, Tamika faced financial hardship. "Cancer bankrupts you," she said, noting that even her "good insurance" eventually reached its maximum. "I remember being down to ten dollars to my name." In addition to her money woes, Tamika was devastated by her weight gain during treatment and its effect on her libido as a single, twenty-five-year-old woman. "I could not imagine ever having sex again, given the stigma of a cancer caused by HPV, and having been asked if I should get an HIV test – and the idea that I'd done something wrong or that it was my fault."

Her cancer diagnosis seemed to take over her life. "There is not a single part of life that cervical cancer doesn't invade. It was just so much in such a short time," she said. "It wrecked me."

> *"There is not a single part of life that cervical cancer doesn't invade. It was just so much in such a short time," she said. "It wrecked me."*

Making Her Cancer Count

It took about two years, Tamika said, "to get my feet back under me." But gradually, she began telling her story, her media background reminding her of the power of her own voice. Rather than giving in to despair, Tamika turned toward sparing other women a similar fate. One of her first forms of advocacy was successfully lobbying the legislature in her home state of Maryland to mandate that insurance companies pay for fertility preservation for young cancer victims – both female and male – an outcome that helped ease her pain. "While it was too late for me, it's so satisfying now to know that other women facing the same heartbreaking situation … will have options I didn't have."

Tamika continued to reach out to other cancer survivors and work on behalf of their struggles. She discovered the power of connection by representing Maryland on a presidential cancer panel, a group that advocates for cancer prevention funding and policies. "In that room, people 'got me.' They understood what it was like to get cancer at a young age. They understood what it was like to struggle to live the rest of my life having had cancer." Through experiences like this, Tamika found a new sense of purpose.

When she started Cervivor in 2005, Tamika had a vision for creating a supportive community of survivors. She decided that if women could find each other online, their voices would be "stronger together" – a message consistent with the core principles of Cervivor. She saw the group working together to collectively dispel myths about cervical cancer. "I believed in the power of women's stories to show that cervical cancer happens to all women. I've seen cervical cancer happen to every type of

person you can think of, and every woman has had to deal with
stigma and shame. I wanted to work toward destroying stigma.
For me, it was a way to continue to make my cancer count."

---

*"I believed in the power of women's stories to show
that cervical cancer happens to all women. I've seen
cervical cancer happen to every type of person you
can think of, and every woman has had to deal with
stigma and shame. I wanted to work toward
destroying stigma. For me, it was a way to
continue to make my cancer count."*

From Support Circle to Juggernaut

Initially, only six women came forward to be featured on
Tamika's website. But, through her hard work and determination, and the willingness of this small group to talk about their
cancer experiences, Cervivor continued to grow. "It took years
and a great deal of work to build trust so that other survivors
could catch the vision of being 'stronger together,'" Tamika
said. Fifteen years later, she channeled Cervivor donations
into Cervivor School, an education program that teaches survivors about cervical cancer prevention, treatment, and advocacy. Cervivor School graduates have gone on to lobby state
legislatures for cervical cancer prevention funding, provide
local or national expertise, and act as advocates on cervical
cancer guideline development. It was through her role in guideline development that I met Tamika.

In speaking with Tamika, I learned that Cervivor community
members most value emotional support as they navigate being
diagnosed and treated, and then living with the disease. Many
Cervivor members called the depth and breadth of connection
with this group lifesaving. There is immense power, these women
say, in being known and understood. The Cervivor network has
gone on to acquire 6,000 members and international reach. It
demonstrates demand for these kinds of support services and

the power of movements generated by the disenfranchised. In fact, some of the most successful and energetic change makers I've encountered are those who struggled, and then rose up, saying, "Enough! I don't want to take it anymore!"

That is my truth in writing this book, my way of mobilizing against tolerance for the status quo. I am simply unwilling to accept so many women dying from a preventable cancer. Tamika, too, has reached her breaking point. "I've known a lot of women who didn't make it. Each of those deaths hurt. Every single one of those lives matters." Tamika turned her own terrible struggle with cervical cancer into something meaningful for herself and others, a narrative echoed again and again by the women I interviewed.

"I've known a lot of women who didn't make it. Each of those deaths hurt. Every single one of those lives matters." Tamika turned her own terrible struggle with cervical cancer into something meaningful for herself and others, a narrative echoed again and again by the women I interviewed.

As I spoke with women across all time zones, above and below the equator, I continued to learn about the role of cervical cancer survivors in founding or adopting organizations – all of them making a difference on an individual, regional, and even global level. I marveled at their courage to reach out as educators and advocates, even while confining their thoughts to their own social media spheres. They see the immense power in spreading the word about cervical cancer, wherever they are in the world, using whatever gifts they have.

Tackling Taboos: What Girls Can't Even Tell Their Mothers

Karla, an engineer by training from Siguatepeque, Honduras, calls herself a reluctant educator (Figure 16.2). Diagnosed with Stage 2B cervical cancer at thirty-five, Karla underwent

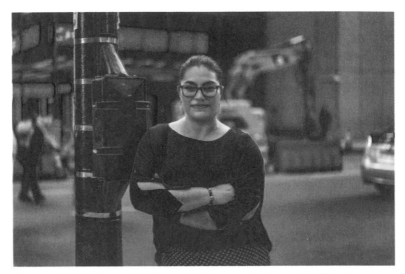

Figure 16.2 Karla, a voice for cervical cancer in her native Honduras

chemotherapy, radiation, and ultimately, a hysterectomy. Then, things got worse. One month after her hysterectomy, Karla coughed and heard a "pop." A week later, she experienced the unwelcome and life-altering complication of stool leaking through her vagina. Karla had developed a fistula (opening) between her intestine and vagina, a condition requiring a colostomy, a surgical diversion of an undamaged piece of the colon into an artificial opening in the abdominal wall. Now dealing with a colostomy and the problems that necessitated it, Karla was not only in physical and emotional pain, she was in social isolation too.

"In Honduras, talking about HPV or sex or cervical cancer – especially a colostomy – is taboo," she said to me. "Girls don't even talk about those things with their mothers." Karla needed support, not stigma, and she found it in Tamika's online support group, Cervivor. Attending Cervivor School helped Karla learn how to talk with others about her experiences openly and knowledgeably. She gradually developed the confidence to be a voice for cervical cancer in Honduras, despite living in a country where discussing female anatomy, HPV, issues related to sex, and colostomies are affronts to cultural norms.

"In Honduras, talking about HPV or sex or cervical cancer – especially a colostomy – is taboo."

Soon Karla was posting information on Facebook about HPV, the HPV vaccine (which Honduras had just started offering to girls between nine and twelve), and cervical cancer screening, and she quickly started fielding followers' questions. Karla gets deep satisfaction from knowledge sharing. "I'm trying to make it normal to talk about sex," she said. "It's not just for those who ask me questions. This work gives me joy and purpose." When stigma threatened to overwhelm her, Karla said, "Enough," and fought back – she channeled her helplessness into the power of contributing to cervical cancer prevention.

"I'm trying to make it normal to talk about sex," she said. "It's not just for those who ask me questions. This work gives me joy and purpose."

Into the Halls of Justice

Some cervical cancer survivors become legislative activists, lobbying for better services, greater awareness, and increased funding for cervical cancer education and prevention. Morgan, the young woman hit with cervical cancer at twenty-four after naively turning down the HPV vaccine as a teenager, has become active about the cause in her Iowa state legislature. By sharing her own story, Morgan and her fellow lobbyists per-suaded the state government of Iowa in December 2019 to declare January a statewide "Cervical Cancer Awareness" month. Iowan legislators agreed, and now the state joins the rest of the country – as well as other countries worldwide – in making the first month of the year a public platform for cervical cancer prevention. Morgan's advocacy has earned her a seat as

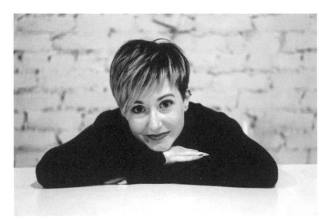

Figure 16.3 Morgan, a state and national advocate. Photo credit: R.K. Anderson.

patient representative on the American Society for Clinical Oncology board, a place at the table during medical guideline developments related to cervical cancer, and one that welcomes her critical perspective on decisions affecting prevention and treatment measures for American women (Figure 16.3).

Morgan has extended her commitment internationally, as well. In partnership with the American Cancer Society, she has been raising money for the construction of Kenya Hope Hostel in Nairobi, which will offer affordable transportation and accommodation for rural Kenyan cervical cancer patients seeking treatment.

Partnering with the Professionals

Cervical cancer sufferers and survivors who want to become advocates already have the necessary information, the passion, and the story. When they join with medical societies, professional forums, or established advocacy groups dedicated to cancer care, they amplify their own voices by offering much-needed insights to professionals and words of inspiration to other persons with cervixes. As a physician and cervical cancer expert, I've had the privilege of "sharing a microphone" with a number of amazing advocates whose experience has greatly deepened my understanding of how to offer cervical cancer patients the highest standard of care.

In Europe, Kim, Denisa, and Icó are outstanding champions for cervical cancer prevention, screening, treatment, and education. Their advocacy has helped thousands of women and it certainly helped me appreciate the power of patient advocacy. Eight years before I met Kim, this Dutch single mother had no idea she would someday devote herself to this cause full-time (Figure 16.4). Kim was diagnosed with cervical cancer at thirty-nine after experiencing minimal bleeding between periods and after she had sex. Kim's children were nine and eleven when she underwent an immediate radical hysterectomy and external and internal radiation. "All I could think was, 'I have to stay alive.' Those were the hardest days."

"All I could think was, 'I have to stay alive.' Those were the hardest days."

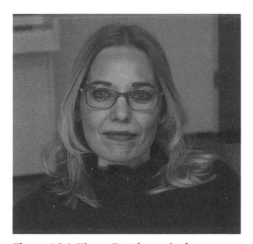

Figure 16.4 Kim, a Dutch cervical cancer survivor and activist

Kim still struggles with lymphedema, skin infections, and a bladder "fried by radiation," as she described it. But she's cancer-free and fierce about HPV vaccination and cervical cancer care. She works for the Salvation Army coordinating peer support and presentations for gynecological cancer patient groups, and is the representative for "Stichting Olijf," the Dutch network for women with gynecological cancers that is part of ENGAGe, the advocacy arm of the European Society of Gynaecological Oncology (ESGO). ESGO is a group of more than 3,400 professionals from across Europe and around the world committed to caring for women with gynecological cancers, and has been dedicated to cervical cancer prevention, research, and education for almost forty years. In 2021, ESGO formed ENGAGe Teens to specifically spread the word to teens about the HPV vaccine and preventing HPV disease.

Kim's fellow ENGAGe representative Denisa, another cervical cancer survivor, has been using the ENGAGe platform to change and educate minds in the Czech Republic (Figure 16.5). "Czech people don't like health care. They have a lot of fear," she

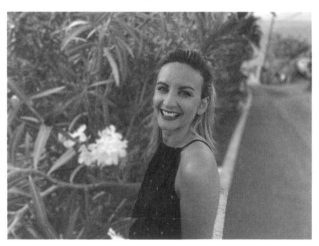

Figure 16.5 Denisa, a cervical cancer survivor and activist from the Czech Republic

explained to me. Denisa, who began bleeding after having sex, wasn't afraid to go to a doctor to investigate her symptoms. Yet when she received a cervical cancer diagnosis at twenty-eight, Denisa was suddenly carrying two burdens: the knowledge she would lose her cervix and the tremendous stigma of her disease.

Denisa described having cervical cancer in the Czech Republic as akin to "wearing a sticker that says, 'I'm promiscuous.' If you have cancer," she said, "you must be doing something wrong."

Denisa described having cervical cancer in the Czech Republic as akin to "wearing a sticker that says, 'I'm promiscuous.' If you have cancer," she said, "you must be doing something wrong." In an effort to combat these perceptions and foster healthy public conversations about cervical cancer, Denisa joined Veronica in 2019 – a gynecological cancer advocacy group in the Czech Republic – which then led her to ENGAGe. She has since been using the platforms of Veronica and ENGAGe to tell anyone who will listen: "HPV causes cervical cancer. It's not genetic. Boys can spread HPV." And that's because, she said, "No one ever told me that."

"Boys can spread HPV." And that's because, she said, "No one ever told me that."

In Hungary, Icó faced similar stigma about her disease (Figure 16.6). Icó was diagnosed with cervical cancer in 2011 after the birth of her second child. Icó's great-grandmother had died of cervical cancer, and while it is not a genetic disease, she was devastated when a CT scan showed a 4.5-centimeter cervical tumor. With a four-year-old and a newborn at home, she received treatment via a radical hysterectomy and thirty external radiation treatments, plus chemotherapy.

Not only was Icó trying to parent while physically and spiritually debilitated, she also felt lonely and isolated during her recovery. "The stigma was pushing me down," she

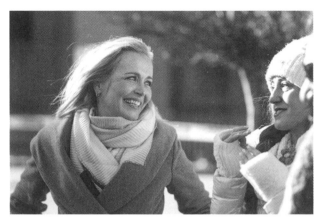

Figure 16.6 Icó, a cervical cancer survivor and activist from Hungary

said. Desperate for connection, Icó did something dramatic: she published her diary and included her email address at the end of it. Now, Icó had connection. "[Women] from every corner of the country contacted me," she marveled. "I was not alone."

Just two years after her diagnosis, Icó and four fellow survivors founded the Malyvavirag Foundation – named after the mallow flower – "unwavering, strong, and beautiful, like us women," she said. This organization then led her to ENGAGe. Icó's vitality is so infectious that she became a featured speaker at the WHO cervical cancer elimination launch in 2020, which is where I met her. "I really believe we can change the world. That we can do this together," she declared. "I love life. It's a big privilege to live."

Icó's vitality is so infectious that she became a featured speaker at the WHO cervical cancer elimination launch in 2020, which is where I met her. "I really believe we can change the world. That we can do this together," she declared. "I love life. It's a big privilege to live."

Combating Stigma with Compassion

Sally Agallo Kwenda, who lives in Nairobi, Kenya, also sees life as a privilege, one repeatedly threatened and hard won (Figure 16.7). In 1999, Sally was diagnosed with AIDS, and suffered not just the terrible physical toll but the emotional scars of learning she'd gotten it from her husband – who had been unfaithful and abandoned her upon her diagnosis. Sally also happened to be pregnant when she was diagnosed with HIV. She had to deal with unexpected preterm labor, which led to the death of her baby. In addition to these ordeals, Sally's burden included social shaming. "In Kenya, life without a child is very difficult," she said. "It is very bad for a woman not to have a child. It is almost as bad as HIV."

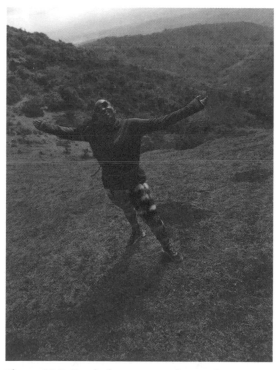

Figure 16.7 Cervical cancer survivor and ostomy patient Sally Agallo Kwenda

"In Kenya, life without a child is very difficult," she said. "It is very bad for a woman not to have a child. It is almost as bad as HIV."

But when PEPFAR and public funding made lifesaving, anti-retroviral treatments available to her in 2013, Sally clawed her way back to life, regaining strength and beating back depression. She began working for MSF (Médecins Sans Frontières or "Doctors Without Borders") as an HIV peer advocate and educator. Her MSF employment granted her first-time access to health insurance, allowing her to get screened for cervical cancer. Then, at thirty-eight, Sally was diagnosed with cervical cancer.

Her insurance enabled her to see a gynecologist, but Sally learned her Stage 2 cancer would require a hysterectomy. Like Tamika, she was devastated to shut the door on childbearing. After her surgery, and with support from friends and colleagues, Sally rebounded once again. She became an advocate – not just for AIDS prevention, but for cervical cancer screening.

When Sally's cancer recurred in her rectum, her doctor told her, "I will give you a colostomy and that will fix your pain." Sally did not know what a colostomy was, and when she woke up: "I found I had intestine hanging outside my body. I was traumatized. No one told me what to expect, or that I would always have to find bags for [the colostomy]." Once again, however, Sally turned challenge into opportunity, this time starting Stoma World Kenya (now Kenya Ostomy Association) to help educate and address the challenges of stoma, including procuring funding for the ostomy bags so hard to find in Kenya.

Despite making strides on behalf of others, Sally still struggles with the cost of dealing with a chronic health problem in a lower-income country. Her job with MSF – and therefore her insurance – ended in 2016. Since then, Sally has been without medical coverage. "I cannot go for checkups – I do not have the money." Yet she remains optimistic and continues to advocate for cervical cancer awareness in Kenya. "I am feeling strong and good, so I think I am okay," she said. "I tell everyone to get screened. I tell every girl who can get the vaccine to get the vaccine. I speak for the American Cancer Society and do the 'Relay for Life.' There is still a lot of stigma here for cervical cancer. The problem is people wait until they have pain or problems to get screened. If I had not gotten screened when I did, I would be dead."

"There is still a lot of stigma here for cervical cancer. The problem is people wait until they have pain or problems to get screened. If I had not gotten screened when I did, I would be dead."

Tech and Ingenuity to the Rescue

Cervical cancer survivors understand their disease better than almost anyone else, making them ingenious advisors when it comes to improving cervical cancer care. I remember talking with Tamika Felder about the "surprise" of a pelvic exam. "Providers do not give women an idea of what it is about or why it is important," she said. To increase the appeal of pelvic exams, Tamika proposed that clinics offer patients introductory videos prior to being examined, making for fewer "surprises" and more open communication between provider and patient. She even suggested making these videos available on cell phones, and thus more readily available to persons with cervixes in lower- and higher-income countries. What a clever, relatively low-tech way to address long-standing emotional barriers to screening.

In New York, cervical cancer survivor Eve is bringing her tech-oriented mind to easing the trauma of cervical cancer treatment. Eve, who was diagnosed with cervical cancer while pregnant at age thirty-three, found her post-delivery, vaginal brachytherapy treatment unbearably painful. "Couldn't this be better?" she asked herself. "Couldn't this be less painful?" Formerly a high-powered Google executive, Eve wasn't used to taking no for an answer. She applied her entrepreneurial savvy toward improving the experience of radiation treatment. She has since been working

with her radiation oncologist Dr. Onyinye Balogun, assistant professor at Weill Cornell Medicine, to develop a gentler form of
radiation equipment eyed for medical mainstream use, a plan
aimed at significantly reducing suffering for future cervical cancer
patients (Figure 16.8).

---

*Eve, who was diagnosed with cervical cancer while
pregnant at age thirty-three, found her post-delivery,
vaginal   brachytherapy   treatment   unbearably
painful. "Couldn't this be better?" she asked herself.
"Couldn't this be less painful?"*

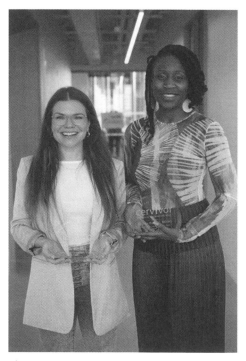

Figure 16.8 Dr. Onyinye Balogun and Eve McDavid first met through Eve's
successful cervical cancer treatment. Together, they are a physician:
patient team who have launched Mission-Driven Tech, a new women's
health venture dedicated to the transformation of gynecologic cancer care
with modern technology. Photo courtesy of Cervivor Inc.

Time to Join the Collective Cry

Cervical cancer survivors are awe inspiring. But we need not endure a brush with this disease to appreciate the growing cries of *Enough!* Those of us lucky enough to be spared cervical cancer are in a unique position: healthy and energetic enough to help persons with cervixes be spared unnecessary death, and free of the day-to-day strain of fighting cancer or worrying about a recurrence. The long-term battle against cervical cancer requires all of us to take part – and most especially, those strong and vital enough to sustain that battle.

How satisfying it is, after all, to serve others simply for the sake of doing so. We get to experience the dual joy of helping women avoid preventable death while experiencing personal fulfillment. Those are the secrets many of us learn when we take part in a cause larger than ourselves, one that allows us to learn and grow in ways we hadn't thought possible.

While some of us may choose to "dive in" to combating cervical cancer by starting our own advocacy projects, it's important to remember that many worthwhile organizations with established initiatives already exist – crying out for greater public involvement. The Reader Resources section at the back of this book lists a wide variety of those organizations, including some not yet mentioned, each supporting strides toward eliminating cervical cancer. Many of these organizations offer creative ways for participants to connect with local fundraising and advocacy efforts – allowing each of us to play a part in the global struggle against cervical cancer.

Perhaps the simplest first step in joining this collective cry of "Enough!" is to choose the person whose story has most inspired or provoked you, and lean in. Look them up. Learn more about them. Follow them on social media. Then think about how you can share their stories with others – face-to-face or through broader media platforms – as a means of generating energy and commitment within yourself as well as others. These small first steps can reverberate quickly into a growing conversation about cervical cancer – allowing for bigger strides toward vanquishing the disease once and for all.

Information Is Fuel for Change

When we share both the cold, hard facts about cervical cancer as well as the intimate stories of real women's lives, we call attention to a cancer frequently relegated to the shadows. We situate cervical cancer front and center; we bring it into the light. We demand that the world stop ignoring a killer. When we share information and stories, we amplify women's voices and push back on fear, stigma, and misinformation. We participate in the future: a world that no longer plays host to the sorrows of cervical cancer.

Each time you make yourself available to talk about cervical cancer – drawing upon what you've learned in this book – you are helping to influence the trajectory of this disease. Instagram, Twitter, Facebook, and TikTok all offer readily accessible ways to address the stigma and shame around cervical cancer, and the Reader Resources section offers plenty of examples and information on how to make the best use of these platforms. You can create your own social media content if you like, but sharing others' voices – the helpful information you find from trusted resources – is a valid and effective way to promote conversations about cervical cancer.

If social media isn't your happy place, pick up your pen and spread the word about cervical cancer in other ways. Consider blogging about the vast numbers of women dying of cervical cancer and what we can do to save them. Consider writing a letter to the editor of a print or online newspaper or magazine about any of the many timely topics and issues discussed in this book. If writing doesn't feel like a good match, consider pitching stories to journalists about the effort to eliminate cervical cancer and encouraging them to engage the public in a long-overdue conversation based on what you've learned so far. When you see misinformation or stigma, speak up. We can all play a role in changing the larger narrative by simply writing or talking about a topic with passion, sincerity, and enlightenment. Even the simple question, "Did you know we can prevent a cancer?" is provocative enough to get the conversation going.

Even the simple question, "Did you know we can prevent a cancer?" is provocative enough to get the conversation going.

Calling All Activists

If you're less of an author and more of an activist, wide-ranging options are available in cervical cancer prevention. In fact, according to New York–based Human Rights Watch, any effort to improve access to HPV vaccination, screening, or treatment makes you more than a cervical cancer advocate – it makes you a *human rights* activist.

In 2018, Human Rights Watch declared it a human right not to die of cervical cancer. Because this cancer is preventable, the declaration stated, all humans should have equal access to the means of preventing it. This bold declaration arose from a Human Rights Watch report affirming the link between health care inequities in the United States and this country's rate and spread of cervical cancer. The report noted the correlation between the limitations on Medicaid access in certain states and subsequent drops in cervical cancer screening rates for those on a low income. Their 2020 follow-up report offered multiple recommendations for preserving the human rights of people with cervixes, including Medicaid expansion to ensure cervical cancer care for low-income patients; improved transportation and expansion of telehealth for women living in rural areas; improved, standardized, HPV-associated cancer education for sixth-graders; and improved training for health workers and policy makers to address the effect of racial bias on cervical cancer prevention.

While these Human Rights Watch initiatives are heartening, these words cannot simply end up buried in reports. These calls to action can morph into prescriptions for change: the chance to tenaciously grasp a human right – the prevention of death from a cancer that need never occur. As readers and fellow believers that women should not die of cervical cancer, know that this template for change exists and is ready to be seized and acted upon.

Dr. Bello, the Nigerian obstetrician, gynecologist, and public health physician concerned with the desperate lack of access to HPV vaccines in her home country, has seized the opportunity to work as a human rights advocate. When she started the RAiSE Foundation in 2015, Dr. Bello's vision was to direct nongovernmental donations toward providing improved medical care, education, and outreach to women and children. She has since capitalized on her position as the First Lady of Niger State to ensure the government requires medical insurance companies to include cervical cancer screening as part of a basic health care package. While she had never experienced cervical cancer, Dr. Bello has felt compelled to tap into her political connections and direct her energies toward stopping the disease on behalf of her fellow humans. When we use our opportunities and strengths and connections for this common purpose, we too become human rights advocates.

Lest these challenges sound daunting, remember: you don't need to be a skilled lobbyist or a health care professional to get started. You don't even need to be particularly "political." Remember, working toward equity in health care means you are working toward human rights. By promoting policies that allow persons with cervixes to access much needed prevention services, we can alleviate suffering and thereby diminish the painful ripple effects of all those connected to the cancer sufferer. That kind of activism is always welcomed.

Teach Your Children Well

Disseminating information about the cause and prevention of cervical cancer is invaluable – and nowhere more so than in the hands of educators. When teachers incorporate this knowledge into a scientific, standardized curriculum, they can arm our children with the tools to dramatically reduce HPV-related cancers and death for themselves and their generation. As parents or concerned citizens, you can directly engage in making this happen. You can start by attending school board meetings or parent-teacher association gatherings and ask what your schools are doing to prevent future suffering from cervical cancer, and you can expand your efforts from there. Whether you are advocating via the state or province or countrywide, within a local school jurisdiction, or even within a school or parent-teacher association, you have the right to ask that children be offered timely education about reproductive health that includes lifesaving information about HPV: how it's spread, its connection to cervical and other cancers, and how it can be circumvented.

The benefits of building this information into school curriculums go beyond the goal of enlightening young minds about preventing cervical cancer and reducing the stigma of HPV. The teachers required to adhere to that curriculum will become better educated and equipped to understand the importance of protecting their reproductive health. Through their children, families of these students will become enlightened about a too-rarely discussed topic. By extension, a whole generation of kids and adults is given the gift of better health. Choosing to work with educators in this way – to spread the word about HPV and its prevention – is a tangible example of making a difference in the cervical cancer elimination strategy directly within your own community. The goodwill behind these efforts will ripple far and wide.

Think before You Vote

In addition to supporting cancer prevention education and lobbying for change in cancer prevention policies, it's critical to consider the implications of who we vote for. We must support representatives focused on furthering the health and well-being of persons with cervixes and of cervical cancer prevention, whether it's at the local level, such as city councils, hospital boards, county commissions, school boards, at stage and regional levels, or on a national scale. We can and should call on our elected officials to value the health of all persons with cervixes.

In addition to supporting cancer prevention education and lobbying for change in cancer prevention policies, it's critical to consider the implications of who we vote for.

When both women and men scrutinize public policy carefully and assess elected officials for their stance on women's health prevention services, we are truly using our power to make a difference. We are supporting a society that can and should prize its women. Beyond focusing on health, we can study how candidates value equity for all, and whether they will work to overcome the patriarchal fabric woven into all our systems, which includes systems of employment, benefit provision, wage-setting, and education about reproductive health, as well as the system that governs women's autonomy over their health care decisions. These actions empower women to seek appropriate health care, including preventative care for cervical cancer. Making women's health care a political priority might seem like a gradual, more indirect way of preventing cervical cancer deaths. But using our votes to elevate women and their health care needs is still a lasting way to make a difference.

A Few More Ideas beyond Authoring and Activism

Sometimes, the best change making happens when we simply "put our bodies on the line." For example, every year in January, the United States recognizes Cervical Cancer Awareness Month. During the lead-up to this event, look for marches and gatherings and fundraisers taking place in January where you can meet other invested allies, develop relationships, and make your presence known to your community.

Make sure you screen for cervical cancer and consider asking a neighbor or friend to come along with you, just like the Teal Sisters do in Zambia.

Bring this book to a book club meeting and discuss cervical cancer and HPV with other book club guests.

Say the word *cervix*. One of the simplest ways to combat stigma is to simply say the words out loud: *cervix*, *vagina*, *cancer*, *Pap smear*. Become more comfortable with talking about these terms with friends and family. Explain to men, in particular, what a speculum is or what screening involves. Talk to friends about screening and vaccination. Let's make cervical cancer as easy to talk about as breast cancer – a disease people rarely talked about out loud until pioneering women and men came along and demanded that breast cancer be openly discussed. By getting on friendlier terms with the words *cervical cancer*, each of us can confront the stigma and stamp out the shame accompanying a cancer that happens to grow on the cervix, at the top of a vagina.

These are simple but effective steps forward. Not all of us are called to be mountain movers, but each of us can be a myth and stigma buster.

Never Underestimate Your Personal Power

Getting to *Enough* will take all of us. Thankfully, we have innumerable ways to get there, and great examples to follow. The women of this book – cancer-sufferers-turned-advocates from across the globe – offer a vision and concrete examples of how each of us can roll up our sleeves and get to work on this cause. We can join Tamika and all the other survivors who take up the torch daily to end this cancer. The need is vast and your efforts count.

As the Cervivor mantra reminds us, "We are stronger together." This is our chance to show how much we believe it.

As the Cervivor mantra reminds us, "We are stronger together." This is our chance to show how much we believe it.

THE CALLING REVISITED

I started this book with the cry, "Enough!" Enough, already. Too many women have faced the scourge of cervical cancer. Too many have seen their lives forever altered. Too many have died senseless deaths. Surely we've gotten to a place now where we've all seen and heard more than enough. Join with me now. Let's declare enough is enough and that it's finally time to act.

I hope it's clear to you by now that cervical cancer, at least in theory, need not exist. The medical community has the knowledge and experience needed to defeat it. We know what causes this cancer, how to detect it, how to treat it, how to prevent it. We can screen for pre-cancer and treat it so early we stop cancer in its tracks. We can find cancer soon enough that it can be treated and cured. We can vaccinate against it and prevent more than 90 percent of all new cases. In the world of cancer, cervical cancer stands alone: it offers us a clear path for preventing it and the very real possibility we can eliminate this disease in our lifetimes.

And yet, as I said at the beginning, I am keenly aware that this task is too big for one person. The onward march of cervical cancer shows no sign of slowing. The suffering and torment and death continue: 340,000 deaths a year. Every year, 600,000 persons with cervixes are diagnosed with cervical cancer. Stopping its murderous rampage will involve all of us.

The world is bombarding this cancer on many fronts. Artificial intelligence promises improved accuracy in VIA testing, the type of screening that lower-income countries essentially rely on but that's moderately reliable as a diagnostic tool.

Definitive HPV-DNA tests are another piece of good news for screening. While the costs of HPV-DNA tests are out of reach in most countries hardest hit by cervical cancer rates, we know that researchers are hard at work on cheaper versions. These versions would require less sophisticated lab processing but offer speedy results with no need for a second visit. The World Health Organization has just approved a new HPV vaccine from China, and India is testing a soon-to-be-available HPV vaccine – developments promising to vanquish the current global supply deficit. The WHO's recent endorsement of a one-dose HPV vaccine addresses not just supply but also cost and logistical issues that continue to plague countries around the world. In 2020, every WHO member country committed to eliminating cervical cancer, offering hope to women everywhere as well as a tremendous opportunity to gather global attention, energy, and political will around a much-neglected, silence-cloaked cause.

Governments, health ministries, institutions, medical societies, NGOs, and nonprofits around the world must take advantage of this moment with planning, persistence, and commitment. And so must you. In the last chapter, I offered many ways ordinary people are joining this courageous and exciting fight – the chance to actually *stop* a cancer – and I hope you will find your place in that tremendous gathering of warriors. In addition to a professional career spent advocating, educating, and caring for patients, writing this book has been my commitment to eliminating cervical cancer. That you will join me, in your own way, is my sincerest hope, and the reason I wrote this book. I hope that you, like some of the survivors in this book, will find *your* voice and make it heard.

My original call for *Enough!* came from a sense of exasperation, from feeling at the end of my rope over women needlessly suffering and dying while everyone around them was losing hope. I had watched for years as political decisions in my own country and abroad left women without access to health care, including cervical cancer vaccination, screening, and treatment. I knew and cared for women-patients directly affected by this lack of care: it caused them tremendous suffering. For some, the absence of sufficient or ongoing care cost their lives. The underlying message was undeniable: the world doesn't value its women. With this realization, I hit an internal tipping point; I was angry and frustrated and outraged. My *Enough!* felt like a cry of despair.

But after talking to so many women and their allies, after learning about so much human ingenuity and capacity for kindness and joy, I've found a different way of saying *Enough!* For me, *Enough!* has morphed into a term of possibility and empowerment. We have *enough* medical knowledge, tests, vaccines, and treatment to prevent women from dying of cancer. We now have *enough* commitment from governments and global health organizations worldwide. We certainly have *enough* models for and examples of cervical cancer being thrust into the spotlight, of brave people and movements throwing off the chains of silence and stigma. And, unquestionably, we have *enough* women willing to come forward with courage to share their stories, to use their voices toward this cause. Their voices are magnificent and worthy of amplifying. Sharing their stories has been a deep privilege for me.

Indeed, the entire journey of writing this book emanates from the power of women and their stories, stories that portray the sheer humanity – the worthiness – of being a person born female. A person who happens to have cervical cancer. Stories tell us that cervical cancer is not just a disease measured by numbers. It is a disease measured by women. Women who laugh, who imagine, who love. Women who hurt, who hope, who call out. Women whose sudden absence creates ripples with concentric circles of loss for everyone in their sphere: children, partners, nieces, cousins, workmates, and dear friends. Losses to communities, workforces, economies, countries, yes. But each of the 341,181 persons with cervixes who died in 2020 possessed a unique spirit and set of gifts. Each left behind a dark hole that can never be filled.

Every sufferer of cervical cancer has a name. You've heard a few of them already: Maria. Tamika. Teolita. Icó. Carol.

Florence. Eve. Karen. Sally. Morgan. Elvira. Kim from the United States and Kim from Amsterdam. Jennifer. Linda. Denisa. Loretta. Barbara. Karla. Emma. Susie. Ruth. Mama. Emily. Angie. Jess. Then there are the names of so many more women who weren't featured in this book. Unimaginably more.

What has happened to every one of them matters.

I hope you are ready to join them and me, to give voice to the *Enough!* in your own heart, however you are able. On behalf of those who have died, enough. On behalf of the persons with cervixes robbed of so much, enough. On behalf of the families and lovers and children, enough. On behalf of our shared humanity, enough. Let's say it together:

> We can rid the world of cervical cancer.
> I can do my part.
> Women are worth it.
> Enough.

ACKNOWLEDGMENTS

As an obstetrician and gynecologist, of course I think of writing a book as a gestation and a birth. And, just as I say about pregnancy and labor … I had no idea what I was in for. Perhaps it is better that way. The travail and the joys reveal themselves along the way.

I have had so many birth attendants for this project.

I will always be thankful to Cami Ostman of the Narrative Project who encouraged me to START while providing valuable online courses to get this new author oriented. I also am indebted to Cami for matching me with my unflappable and "perfect for me" book coach Dana Tye Rally. Coach Dana expertly guided me as we put structure behind the beast, provided innumerable (and I do mean innumerable) chapter edits for refinement, cajoled me with statements like "I think I am going to have to kill you if you don't quit writing like a professor," and showered me with humor over three years of near-weekly rounds of revisions and Zoom meetings. Dana, I think I will always carry your voice in my head – and that is a good thing! I could not have written this book without the brilliant research skills of McKenna Tennant and Annalivia Robinson. Your tireless searching and cataloging of studies into beautiful research notes, combined with the energy and dedication you brought to this project despite having "day jobs," allowed me to put teeth into the text as I crafted chapters. You are strong and wise beyond your years. And then there was the "closer": Sara DeBoer. Your incisive ability to combine chapters, refine sentences, create subtitles, and wield a scalpel while dissecting text sharpened the manuscript immensely and brought us closer to the final birth. Sara, your enthusiasm and witty suggestions rescued me repeatedly. I am beyond grateful. May others come to know your editing prowess.

My agents Laura Bardolph and David Bratt of BBH Literary who took me on ... bless you! ... you shepherded me as a neophyte through the stressful process of book proposals and submissions – and gave me hope by believing in this project. Thank you for your persistence!

And to Anna Whiting, Camille Lee-Own, and Laura Simmons – my editing and production team, Josh Hamel and Jasmine Short in marketing, and all the great behind-the-scenes individuals at Cambridge University Press – you took a chance on a first-time author and immediately grabbed the vision and hope for moving the needle toward greater equity in health care for all who have cervixes. Your helpful suggestions, teamwork, and confidence in the project sustained and energized me as the birth of the book came closer to the finish line and I was struggling with third trimester fatigue.

I could never have written this book if my career in obstetrics and gynecology and global health had not been inspired and fostered by so many. To the myriad individuals across continents and organizations with whom I have been privileged to work – your passion frequently challenged me to ask hard questions, and you've modeled health equity and justice through your contributions via research, service, policy development, and advocacy. A special thank you to those who gave up your time to be interviewed for this book, most of whom I could not specifically name in these pages. Please know your wisdom is embedded in the text. To my department chairs at the University of Washington, Dr. Eschenbach, who allowed me a sabbatical at the World Health Organization in 2009 – a season that served as the impetus for so many professional opportunities – and

Dr. Goff, who allowed me a year off in 2020 when I said, "I want to write a book," I thank you both for your leadership and flexibility. To my colleagues in our department of Obstetrics & Gynecology, I could not have pursued my professional passions without your generous spirits and willingness to cover my patient care responsibilities so I could work in Geneva, or countries like Namibia or Malawi. I am especially indebted to my partners at Harborview. You have inspired me relentlessly over thirty years. What a privilege to serve patients together in a clinic and hospital that walks the talk of offering top-notch health care to all – regardless of social indicators.

To my spiritual support crew – we have raised babies, buried parents, wrestled with Faith, and traveled our adulthoods together. I cannot thank you enough. You lifted me up always, even when the lifting was heavy. You are the true embodiment of Community.

To my three BOYS. Buckley – my life partner – the smartest thing ever was marrying you thirty-six years ago. Thank you for having my back, always, as we've shared our ups and downs for decades. Your patience and support have been unwavering over these past three years as I ignored you countless evenings and weekends and disappeared for weeks at a time to write. Thank you for cooking and caring for me – and for always sharing your laugh, which remains, hands down, one of my favorite things in life.

Conor and Shane – my sons – you offered encouragement and told me I could finish this book even when I did not think it was possible. Over the years, you have celebrated successes and generously listened to SO MANY stories about reproductive health care and the power of women! Thank you for both for your fierceness and for being feminists. I could not be more proud of the men you are.

And lastly, to those who truly gave me the reason to write this book: the individuals who have honored me by calling me your physician, and to those who took a chance on telling a perfect stranger your cancer journey. Thank you is not *Enough* – but know I will always carry you in my core.

READER RESOURCES

American Indian Cancer Foundation

www.americanindiancancer.org

Native Americans govern this national nonprofit described in Chapter 14. The organization was created to address Indigenous communities in the United States shouldering a disproportionate share of the cancer burden. The site's section on cervical cancer features culturally tailored information, population-specific data for policy makers and community strategists, shareable infographics, and stories from cervical cancer survivors.

Cervivor

https://cervivor.org

Tamika Felder, who shared her story of surviving cervical cancer in this book, founded Cervivor through her commitment to supporting and openly discussing women's experiences with the disease. The manifesto for this patient advocacy group talks about ending shame and raising awareness: *No more whispering. No more suffering. No more women dying!* It embraces the survivor community through a program known as "Cervivor School," which trains cervical cancer survivors to act as ambassadors and to share their stories on the Cervivor site, YouTube channel (CervivorTV), and face-to-face in their communities.

ENGAGe (European Network of Gynaecological Cancer Advocacy Groups)

www.engage.esgo.org

ENGAGe represents a network of European patient advocacy groups – seventy-six from thirty European countries – working in concert with the European Society of Gynaecological Oncology to educate the public and empower women dealing with gynecological cancers, including cervical cancer. Among its projects are ongoing "patient advocacy seminars," which highlight the experiences of such patient advocates as Icó, Denisa, and Kim, who shared their stories in Chapter 16. ENGAGe also features a specific branch for youth: the ENGAGe Teens Project supports increased awareness of HPV and the HPV vaccine among teenage girls and their peers.

Gavi

www.gavi.org

Gavi, the Vaccine Alliance, was founded to support equitable access to health- and life-giving vaccines to countries across the world. In the effort to end cervical cancer, Gavi has played a key role in ensuring the world's lowest-income countries attain access to the HPV vaccine. Gavi possesses a considerable global reach through its partnerships with powerful organizations such as the World Health Organization, UNICEF, the World Bank, and the Bill & Melinda Gates Foundation, and it continues to welcome like-minded partnerships of all kinds.

The Global Initiative Against HPV and Cervical Cancer

www.giahc.org

U.S. gynecologist Dr. Shobha Krishnan is the founder and leader of this global group that aligns itself with the effort to eliminate cervical cancer worldwide. The group works in partnership with nonprofits, academic institutions, and governments in a broad array of efforts ranging from research to advocacy. The group also worked with the Global Film Fund to produce and distribute *Lady Ganga: Nilza's Story* (www.ladyganga.world), featuring cervical cancer sufferer Michele Baldwin's journey (see Chapter 14) down the Ganges River of India to raise awareness about the disease.

Grounds for Health

www.groundsforhealth.org

Grounds for Health began through a partnership between an American businessman and a retired doctor who took a trip to source coffee in Huatusco, Mexico, and discovered the shocking cervical cancer death rate of women working in local coffee cooperatives. This internationally respected nonprofit now works in partnership with these coffee cooperatives, along with local health organizations and local NGOs across Latin America and Africa, to improve supply of and access to cervical cancer prevention services for workers in the coffee industry, as well as those working in tea, flower, and cocoa production.

Human Rights Watch

www.hrw.org

This investigative advocacy group has researched and produced two excellent reports on the failure to equitably address cervical cancer in the United States: "'We Need Access': Ending Preventable Deaths from Cervical Cancer in Rural Georgia" (2020) and "It Should Not Happen: Alabama's Failure to Prevent Cervical Cancer Death in the Black Belt" (2018). These reports helped raise awareness of the dire lack of access to cervical cancer prevention and treatment services within marginalized regions of a higher-income country. Both reports are searchable using the site's "Reports" link and offer tangible ways to engage in activism with a focus on cervical cancer.

Jo's Cervical Cancer Trust

www.jostrust.org.uk

Considered the United Kingdom's leading cervical cancer charity, Jo's Cervical Cancer Trust provides trustworthy information and support for patients worldwide through its website and sponsors ongoing, UK-based campaigns for disease awareness, prevention, and treatment. The group envisions a future without cervical cancer. It offers opportunities to donate to its research and policy work, volunteer locally in its awareness-raising campaigns, and act as ambassadors in promoting the group's mission.

Kenya Ostomy Association

http://kenyaostomyassociation.com

Sally Agallo Kwenda, another cervical cancer survivor highlighted in Chapter 16, founded this organization as a means of providing essential information and support to patients living with ileostomies, urostomies, and colostomies in Kenya and East Africa, many of whom would otherwise lack access to the services required to manage this condition. This patient-led organization also works in support of cancer prevention and includes awareness-raising ambassadors to advocate for its representatives worldwide.

Mission-Driven Tech

www.missiondriventech.com

Cervical cancer survivor Eve McDavid, the former Google executive featured in Chapter 16, cofounded the Mission-Driven Tech initiative after a particularly traumatic experience with brachytherapy treatment. She and her cofounder, radiation oncologist and Weill Cornell Medicine Assistant Professor Dr. Onyinye Balogun, are working toward transforming gynecological cancer care, starting with the design of newer, better-fitting brachytherapy devices to reduce discomfort and side effects associated with radiation treatment for diseases such as cervical cancer while improving the effectiveness of these treatments overall.

Navegación de Pacientes Internacional

www.npint.org/en/home/

This Latin American–based organization was created to work with Spanish-speaking cancer patients to help them navigate through the health care system, particularly in regions of the continent struggling with equitable access to these services. Honduran patient-advocate and cervical cancer survivor Karla Chavez, who appeared in Chapter 16, works with this organization. Navegación de Pacientes Internacional trains volunteers directly to offer these services throughout Latin America and welcomes donations and support worldwide.

Organization of African First Ladies for Development

www.oaflad.org

More than twenty years ago, thirty-seven wives of African national leaders formed this proactive health care organization. The group's members are committed to promoting policy change, social awareness, and mobilization of resources in support of maternal and infant health, including vaccination against HPV. In addition to advocating for services to reduce Africa's distressingly high rates of cervical cancer, the African

First Ladies Organization raises awareness and supports initiatives that address the continent's ongoing HIV and AIDS pandemic.

RAiSE Foundation

www.raisefoundation.org.ng

This Nigerian-based organization, founded by obstetrician gynecologist Dr. Amina Abubakar Bello, offers practical, on-the-ground interventions in maternal and infant health, including free screenings for cervical cancer and breast cancer, the prevention and treatment of fistulas, advocacy for the education of girls, and vocational training for women. The group's endorsement of the global initiative to eliminate cervical cancer is consistent with their motto: "Healthy Woman, Healthy Nation," which supports the belief that when a community works in concert to raise the health and education levels of its women, everyone benefits.

Teal Sisters Foundation

https://www.tealsistersfoundation.org

Cervical cancer survivor Karen Nakawala, the founder of the Teal Sisters Foundation described in Chapter 14, continues to parlay her background as a Zambian radio and television celebrity into encouraging group members to speak openly and comfortably about their experiences with the disease. Originally based in Zambia, the Teal Sisters have expanded to serving patients and survivors in many African countries, offering not only community education and fellowship but also desperately needed physical and financial support for cervical cancer patients. Their outreach programs include cervical screening for women in prison and funding for women forced to leave their homes for cancer treatment in the capital city of Lusaka, currently Zambia's only radiation treatment facility.

TogetHER for Health

https://togetherforhealth.org

This U.S.-based organization funds and implements evidence-based programs in lower-income countries with the singular goal of ending cervical cancer. U.S. readers may be especially interested in the current efforts of "Operation Wipe Out," an Alabama-based initiative aimed at eliminating cervical cancer in this southern state, which loses almost 50 percent more persons with cervixes to the disease than anywhere else in the country. To donate to this organization, visit https://secure.givelively.org /donate/panorama.

World Health Organization Cervical Cancer Elimination Initiative

www.who.int/initiatives/cervical-cancer-elimination-initiative

As the agency responsible for the promotion of public health among the world's most vulnerable, the World Health Organization secured in 2020 the support of all 194 members of the United Nations, who agreed to ratify this groundbreaking global initiative against a woman-only cancer. The initiative lays out a plan for ending cervical cancer worldwide within the next century and offers a powerful endorsement and incentive for all organizations – be they established or grassroots groups – to align themselves with this global mission.

REFERENCES

Chapter 1

1. OECD and World Health Organization. *Health at a Glance: Asia/Pacific 2020*. 2020. https://doi.org/10.1787/26b007cd-en www.oecdilibrary.org/content/publication/26b007cd-en

Chapter 2

1. Koutsky, L. A., K. A. Ault, C. M. Wheeler, *et al.* "A Controlled Trial of a Human Papillomavirus Type 16 Vaccine." [In Eng]. *N Engl J Med* **347**, no. 21 (Nov 21, 2002): 1645–51. https://doi.org/10.1056/NEJMoa020586
2. World Health Organization. *Global Strategy to Accelerate the Elimination of Cervical Cancer as a Public Health Problem*. World Health Organization, 17 November 2020. Global Strategy.

Chapter 3

1. World Health Organization. *Global Strategy to Accelerate the Elimination of Cervical Cancer as a Public Health Problem*. World Health Organization, 17 November 2020. Global Strategy.

Chapter 4

1. Kim, G. "Harald zur Hausen's Experiments on Human Papillomavirus Causing Cervical Cancer (1976–1987)." *Embryo Project Encyclopedia*, 2017. ISSN: 1940–5030. http://embryo.asu.edu/handle/10776/11444
2. Winer, R. L., S. K. Lee, J. P. Hughes, *et al.* "Genital Human Papillomavirus Infection: Incidence and Risk Factors in a Cohort of

Female University Students." *Am J Epidemiol* **157**, no. 3 (Feb 1, 2003): 218–26. https://doi.org/10.1093/ajc/kwf180

3. *Genital HPV Infection – Basic Fact Sheet*. Division of STD Prevention, National Center for HIV, Viral Hepatitis, STD, and TB Prevention, Centers for Disease Control and Prevention, 2022. Accessed Jan 10, 2023. www.cdc.gov/std/hpv/hpv-Fs-July-2017.pdf

4. Winer, R. L., J. P. Hughes, Q. Feng, *et al.* "Condom Use and the Risk of Genital Human Papillomavirus Infection in Young Women." *N Engl J Med* **354**, no. 25 (Jun 22, 2006): 2645–54. https://doi.org/10.1056/NEJMoa053284. www.ncbi.nlm.nih.gov/pubmed/16790697

5. Koutsky, L. A., K. K. Holmes, C. W. Critchlow, *et al.* "A Cohort Study of the Risk of Cervical Intraepithelial Neoplasia Grade 2 or 3 in Relation to Papillomavirus Infection." *N Engl J Med* **327**, no. 18 (Oct 29, 1992): 1272–8. https://doi.org/10.1056/NEJM199210293271804 www.ncbi.nlm.nih.gov/pubmed/1328880

6. Tartaglia, E., K. Falasca, J. Vecchiet, *et al.* "Prevalence of HPV Infection among HIV-Positive and HIV-Negative Women in Central/Eastern Italy: Strategies of Prevention." *Oncol Lett* **14**, no. 6 (Dec 2017): 7629–35. https://doi.org/10.3892/ol.2017.7140

Chapter 5

1. Haelle, T. "The Great Success and Enduring Dilemma of Cervical Cancer Screening." NPR, 2015. www.npr.org/sections/health-shots/2015/04/30/398872421/the-great-success-and-enduring-dilemma-of-cervical-cancer-screening

2. Wang, W., E. Arca, A. Sinha, *et al.* "Cervical Cancer Screening Guidelines and Screening Practices in 11 Countries: A Systematic Literature Review." *Prev Med Rep* **28** (Aug 2022): 101813. https://doi.org/10.1016/j.pmedr.2022.101813 www.ncbi.nlm.nih.gov/pubmed/35637896

3. Yang, D. X., P. R. Soulos, B. Davis, C. P. Gross, and J. B. Yu. "Impact of Widespread Cervical Cancer Screening: Number of Cancers Prevented and Changes in Race-Specific Incidence." *Am J Clin Oncol* **41**, no. 3 (Mar 2018): 289–94. https://doi.org/10.1097/COC.0000000000000264 www.ncbi.nlm.nih.gov/pubmed/26808257

4. St. Laurent, J., R. Luckett, and S. Feldman. "HPV Vaccination and the Effects on Rates of HPV-Related Cancers." *Curr Probl Cancer* **42**, no. 5 (Sep 2018): 493–506. https://doi.org/10.1016/j.currproblcancer .2018.06.004 www.ncbi.nlm.nih.gov/pubmed/30041818

5. "HPV Cancers." Human Papillomavirus (HPV), Centers for Disease Control and Prevention (CDC), 2022. Accessed Jan 10, 2023. www.cdc.gov/hpv/parents/cancer.html

6. Schnatz, P. F., K. E. Sharpless, and D. M. O'Sullivan. "Use of Human Papillomavirus Testing in the Management of Atypical Glandular Cells." *J Low Genit Tract Dis* **13**, no. 2 (Apr 2009): 94–101. https://doi .org/10.1097/LGT.0b013e318183a438 www.ncbi.nlm.nih.gov /pubmed/19387129

7. Zeferino, L. C., S. H. Rabelo-Santos, L. L. Villa, *et al.* "Value of HPV-DNA Test in Women with Cytological Diagnosis of Atypical Glandular Cells (AGC)." *Eur J Obstet Gynecol Reprod Biol* **159**, no. 1 (Nov 2011): 160–4. https://doi.org/10.1016/j.ejogrb.2011.05.023 www.ncbi.nlm.nih.gov/pubmed/21680079

8. Gage, J. C., M. Schiffman, H. A. Katki, *et al*, "Reassurance against Future Risk of Precancer and Cancer Conferred by a Negative Human Papillomavirus Test." *J Natl Cancer Inst* **106**, no. 8 (Aug 2014): dju153. https://doi.org/10.1093/jnci/dju153 www.ncbi.nlm.nih.gov /pubmed/25038467

9. Dillner, J., M. Rebolj, P. Birembaut, *et al.* "Long Term Predictive Values of Cytology and Human Papillomavirus Testing in Cervical Cancer Screening: Joint European Cohort Study." *BMJ* **337** (Oct 13, 2008): a1754. https://doi.org/10.1136/bmj.a1754 www.ncbi.nlm.nih .gov/pubmed/18852164

Chapter 6

1. Mohamed, S. M., T. Aagaard, L. U. Fokdal, *et al.* "Assessment of Radiation Doses to the Para-Aortic, Pelvic, and Inguinal Lymph Nodes Delivered by Image-Guided Adaptive Brachytherapy in Locally Advanced Cervical Cancer." *Brachytherapy* **14**, no. 1 (Jan-Feb 2015): 56–61. https://doi.org/10.1016/j.brachy.2014.07.005 www .ncbi.nlm.nih.gov/pubmed/25176182

2. Kuku, S., C. Fragkos, M. McCormack, and A. Forbes. "Radiation-Induced Bowel Injury: The Impact of Radiotherapy on Survivorship after Treatment for Gynaecological Cancers." *Br J Cancer* **109**, no. 6 (Sep 17, 2013): 1504–12. https://doi.org/10.1038/bjc.2013.491 www.ncbi.nlm .nih.gov/pubmed/24002603

3. "Behind the Screen: Revealing the True Cost of Cervical Cancer." Jo's Trust, 2014. Accessed Jan 10, 2023. www.jostrust.org.uk/get-involved/campaign-0/behind-screen

Chapter 7

1. "HIV Key Facts." World Health Organization, 2022. Accessed Jan 10, 2023. www.who.int/news-room/fact-sheets/detail/hiv-aids

2. "Global HIV & Aids Statistics – Fact Sheet." UNAIDS, 2021. Accessed Jan 10, 2023. www.unaids.org/en/resources/fact-sheet

3. Stelzle, D., L. F. Tanaka, K. K. Lee, *et al.* "Estimates of the Global Burden of Cervical Cancer Associated with HIV." *Lancet Glob Health* **9**, no. 2 (Feb 2021): e161–e69. https://doi.org/10.1016/S2214-109X(20) 30459-9 www.ncbi.nlm.nih.gov/pubmed/33212031

4. Liu, G., M. Sharma, N. Tan, and R. V. Barnabas. "HIV-Positive Women Have Higher Risk of Human Papilloma Virus Infection, Precancerous Lesions, and Cervical Cancer." *AIDS* **32**, no. 6 (Mar 27, 2018): 795–808. https://doi.org/10.1097/QAD.0000000000001765 www.ncbi.nlm.nih.gov/pubmed/29369827

5. Massad, L. S., X. Xie, R. Burk, *et al.* "Long-Term Cumulative Detection of Human Papillomavirus among HIV Seropositive Women." *AIDS* **28**, no 17 (Nov 13, 2014): 2601–8. https://doi.org/10.1097/QAD .0000000000000455 www.ncbi.nlm.nih.gov/pubmed/25188771

6. Rowhani-Rahbar, A., S. E. Hawes, P. S. Sow, *et al.* "The Impact of HIV Status and Type on the Clearance of Human Papillomavirus Infection among Senegalese Women." *J Infect Dis* **196**, no. 6 (Sep 15, 2007): 887–94, https://doi.org/10.1086/520883 www.ncbi.nlm.nih .gov/pubmed/17703420

7. Greene, S. A., H. De Vuyst, G. C. John-Stewart, *et al.* "Effect of Cryotherapy vs Loop Electrosurgical Excision Procedure on Cervical Disease Recurrence among Women with HIV and High-Grade Cervical Lesions in Kenya: A Randomized Clinical Trial." *JAMA* **322**,

no. 16 (Oct 22, 2019): 1570–79. https://doi.org/10.1001/jama
.2019.14969 www.ncbi.nlm.nih.gov/pubmed/31638680

8. "HIV Prevalence among Adults (15–49)." UNAIDS, 2021. Accessed
April 2, 2021. https://aidsinfo.unaids.org/

9. Yimer, N. B., M. A. Mohammed, K. Solomon, *et al.* "Cervical Cancer
Screening Uptake in Sub-Saharan Africa: A Systematic Review and
Meta-Analysis." *Public Health* **195** (Jun 2021): 105–11. https://doi.org
/10.1016/j.puhe.2021.04.014 www.ncbi.nlm.nih.gov/pubmed/
34082174

10. "Adolescents and Youth Dashboard." United Nations Population
Fund. Accessed Jan 10, 2023. www.unfpa.org/data/dashboard/
adolescent-youth

11. Petroni, S., R. Yates, M. Siddiqui, *et al.* "Understanding the
Relationships between HIV and Child Marriage: Conclusions from
an Expert Consultation." *Adolescent Health* **64**, no. 6 (2019): 694–96.
https://doi.org/https://doi.org/10.1016/j.jadohealth.2019.02.001

12. Mugo, N. R., R. Heffron, D. Donnell, *et al.* "Increased Risk of HIV-1
Transmission in Pregnancy: A Prospective Study among African
HIV-1-Serodiscordant Couples." *AIDS* **25**, no. 15 (Sep 24, 2011):
1887–95. https://doi.org/10.1097/QAD.0b013e32834a9338 www
.ncbi.nlm.nih.gov/pubmed/21785321

13. "2023 World Population by Country." World Population Review.
2023. Accessed Jan 10, 2023. https://worldpopulationreview.com/
country-rankings/birth-rate-by-country

14. Thomson, K. A., J. Hughes, J. M. Baeten, *et al.* "Increased Risk of HIV
Acquisition among Women throughout Pregnancy and during the
Postpartum Period: A Prospective Per-Coital-Act Analysis among
Women with HIV-Infected Partners." *J Infect Dis* **218**, no. 1 (Jun 5,
2018): 16–25, https://doi.org/10.1093/infdis/jiy113 www
.ncbi.nlm.nih.gov/pubmed/29514254

15. "Global Health Go Further: Saving Women's Lives from Cervical
Cancer in Sub-Saharan Africa." George W. Bush Presidential
Center, 2022. www.bushcenter.org/topics/global-health/go-further

16. Westrich, J. A., C. J. Warren, and D. Pyeon. "Evasion of Host
Immune Defenses by Human Papillomavirus." *Virus Res* **231** (Mar 2,
2017): 21–33. https://doi.org/10.1016/j.virusres.2016.11.023 www
.ncbi.nlm.nih.gov/pubmed/27890631

17. Williams, V. M., M. Filippova, U. Soto, and P. J. Duerksen-Hughes. "HPV-DNA Integration and Carcinogenesis: Putative Roles for Inflammation and Oxidative Stress." *Future Virol* **6**, no. 1 (Jan 1, 2011): 45–57. https://doi.org/10.2217/fvl.10.73 www.ncbi.nlm.nih.gov/pubmed/21318095

Chapter 8

1. Gossa, W., and M. D. Fetters. "How Should Cervical Cancer Prevention Be Improved in LMICs?" *AMA J Ethics* **22**, no. 2 (Feb 1, 2020): E126–34. https://doi.org/10.1001/amajethics.2020.126 www.ncbi.nlm.nih.gov/pubmed/32048583
2. "Leading Cancers by Age, Sex, Race and Ethnicity." United States Cancer Statistics: Data Visualizations, Centers for Disease Control and Prevention, 2019. Accessed Jan 10, 2023. https://gis.cdc.gov/Cancer/USCS/#/Demographics/
3. Kelly, J. J., A. P. Lanier, T. Schade, *et al.* "Cancer Disparities among Alaska Native People, 1970–2011." *Prev Chronic Dis* **11** (2014): E221. https://doi.org/10.5888/pcd11.130369 http://dx.doi.org/10.5888/pcd11.130369
4. Datta, G. D., M.-H. Mayrand, and B. A. Glenn. "Correspondence on the Increasing Incidence of Stage IV Cervical Cancer in the USA: What Factors Are Related?" *Int J Gynecol Cancer* **33** (Jan 3, 2023): 136. https://doi.org/10.1136/ijgc-2022-004066 www.ncbi.nlm.nih.gov/pubmed/36307146
5. Ford, S., W. Tarraf, K. P. Williams, L. A. Roman, and R. Leach. "Differences in Cervical Cancer Screening and Follow-Up for Black and White Women in the United States." *Gynecol Oncol* **160**, no. 2 (Feb 2021): 369–74. https://doi.org/10.1016/j.ygyno.2020.11.027 www.ncbi.nlm.nih.gov/pubmed/33323276
6. "Cancer Stat Facts: Cervical Cancer." National Cancer Institute: Surveillance, Epidemiology, and End Results Program, 2019. https://seer.cancer.gov/statfacts/html/cervix.html
7. "Cervical Cancer: Statistics." Cancer.net, 2022. www.cancer.net/cancer-types/cervical-cancer/statistics
8. Watson, M., V. Benard, C. Thomas, *et al.* "Cervical Cancer Incidence and Mortality among American Indian and Alaska Native Women,

1999–2009." *Am J Public Health* **104**, Suppl 3 (Jun 2014): S415–22.
https://doi.org/10.2105/AJPH.2013.301681 www.ncbi.nlm.nih.gov/
pubmed/24754650

9. Farley, J. H., J. F. Hines, R. R. Taylor, *et al.* "Equal Care Ensures Equal
Survival for African-American Women with Cervical Carcinoma."
Cancer **91**, no. 4 (Feb 15, 2001): 869–73. www.ncbi.nlm.nih.gov/
pubmed/11241257

10. Shannon, G. D., O. H. Franco, J. Powles, Y. Leng, and N. Pashayan.
"Cervical Cancer in Indigenous Women: The Case of Australia."
Maturitas **70**, no. 3 (Nov 2011): 234–45. https://doi.org/10.1016/j
.maturitas.2011.07.019 www.ncbi.nlm.nih.gov/pubmed/21889857

11. Usera-Clavero, M., D. Gil-Gonzalez, D. La Parra-Casado, *et al.*
"Inequalities in the Use of Gynecological Visits and Preventive
Services for Breast and Cervical Cancer in Roma Women in Spain."
Int J Public Health **65**, no. 3 (Apr 2020): 273–80. https://doi.org/10
.1007/s00038-019-01326-w www.ncbi.nlm.nih.gov/pubmed/
31938808

12. Yu, L., S. A. Sabatino, and M. C. White. "Rural-Urban and Racial/
Ethnic Disparities in Invasive Cervical Cancer Incidence in the
United States, 2010–2014." *Prev Chronic Dis* **16** (Jun 6 2019): E70.
https://doi.org/10.5888/pcd16.180447 www.ncbi.nlm.nih.gov/
pubmed/31172917

13. Srivastava, A., J. M. Barnes, S. Markovina, J. K. Schwarz, and
P. W. Grigsby. "The Impact of the Closure of Women's Health Clinics
on Cervical Cancer in the United States." *Int J Radiat Oncol Biol Phys*
105, no. 1 (2019): S98. https://doi.org/10.1016/j.ijrobp.2019.06.581

14. Boom, K., M. Lopez, M. Daheri, *et al.* "Perspectives on Cervical
Cancer Screening and Prevention: Challenges Faced by Providers
and Patients along the Texas–Mexico Border." *Perspect Public Health*
139, no. 4 (Jul 2019): 199–205. https://doi.org/10.1177/
1757913918793443 www.ncbi.nlm.nih.gov/pubmed/30117782

15. Crary, D. "Republicans Are Succeeding in a State-by-State Strategy
to Defund Planned Parenthood." Associated Press, 2016. www
.businessinsider.com/ap-state-by-state-strategy-wielded-to-defund-
planned-parenthood–2016-3

16. Crawford, J., F. Ahmad, D. Beaton, and A. S. Bierman. "Cancer Screening Behaviours among South Asian Immigrants in the UK, US and Canada: A Scoping Study." *Health Soc Care Community* **24**, no. 2 (Mar 2016): 123–53. https://doi.org/10.1111/hsc.12208 www.ncbi.nlm.nih.gov/pubmed/25721339

17. Wentzensen, N., M. A. Clarke, and R. B. Perkins. "Impact of COVID-19 on Cervical Cancer Screening: Challenges and Opportunities to Improving Resilience and Reduce Disparities." *Prev Med* **151** (Oct 2021): 106596. https://doi.org/10.1016/j.ypmed.2021.106596 www.ncbi.nlm.nih.gov/pubmed/34217415

18. Ivanus, U., T. Jerman, U. Gasper Oblak, *et al.* "The Impact of the COVID-19 Pandemic on Organised Cervical Cancer Screening: The First Results of the Slovenian Cervical Screening Programme and Registry." *Lancet Reg Health Eur* **5** (Jun 2021): 100101. https://doi.org/10.1016/j.lanepe.2021.100101 www.ncbi.nlm.nih.gov/pubmed/34557821

19. "Cancer Screening & COVID-19." American Cancer Society, 2022. www.cancer.org/healthy/find-cancer-early/cancer-screening-during-covid-19-pandemic.html

20. De Sanjosé, S. "Restarting Cervical Screening Programs during and after the COVID-19 Pandemic." HPV World. www.hpvworld.com/articles/restarting-cervical-screening-programs-during-and-after-the-covid-19-pandemic/

Chapter 9

1. Abbas, K. M., K. van Zandvoort, M. Brisson, and M. Jit. "Effects of Updated Demography, Disability Weights, and Cervical Cancer Burden on Estimates of Human Papillomavirus Vaccination Impact at the Global, Regional, and National Levels: A Prime Modelling Study." *Lancet Glob Health* **8**, no. 4 (Apr 2020): e536-e44. https://doi.org/10.1016/S2214-109X(20)30022-X www.ncbi.nlm.nih.gov/pubmed/32105613

2. "WHO HPV Vaccine Global Market Study, April 2022." WHO, 2022. Accessed Jan 14, 2023. www.who.int/publications/m/item/who-hpv-vaccine-global-market-study-april–2022

3. "WHO Global Market Study: HPV." www.who.int/immunization/ programmes_systems/procurement/mi4a/platform/module2/ WHO_HPV_market_study_public_summary_Dec2019.pdf?ua=1 Accessed April 8, 2021. The original 2019 global HPV vaccine market study is no longer available on the World Health Organization website. However, the updated HPV vaccine Global Market Study, from April 2022 (Ref. 9.2) does state that "affordability remains a concern for middle-income countries that are no longer or never were supported by Gavi or the PAHO revolving fund" (p. 6, accessed Jan 14, 2023).

4. "Namibia: Human Papillomavirus and Related Cancers, Fact Sheet 2023." ICO/IARC Information Centre on HPV and Cancer, 2023. Accessed May 6, 2023. https://hpvcentre.net/statistics/reports/ NAM_FS.pdf

5. "Namibia to Introduce HPV Vaccine to Teenagers for Cervical Cancer Prevention." *The Star*, 2022. Accessed March 5, 2023. www .thestar.com.my/news/world/2022/11/04/namibia-to-introduce-hpv-vaccine-to-teenagers-for-cervical-cancer-prevention

6. "New World Bank Country Classifications by Income Level: 2022–2023." World Bank, 2022. Accessed Jan 14, 2023. https:// blogs.worldbank.org/opendata/new-world-bank-country-classifications-income-level-2022-2023

7. Slobin, J. "How Much Does a Flu Shot Cost without Insurance in 2021?" Talk to Mira, 2022. Accessed Jan 14, 2023. https://www .talktomira.com/post/how-much-is-a-flu-shot-with-or-without-insurance

8. "CDC Vaccine Price List." Vaccines for Children Program (VFC), Centers for Disease Control and Prevention (CDC), updated Jan 1, 2023. Accessed Jan 14, 2023. www.cdc.gov/vaccines/programs/vfc/ awardees/vaccine-management/price-list/index.html

9. "Meeting of the Strategic Advisory Group of Experts on Immunization, October 2019: Conclusions and Recommendations." *Wkly Epidemiol Rec* **94**, no. 47 (Nov 22, 2019): 541–60. https://reliefweb.int/report/world/weekly-epidemiological-record-wer-22-november-2019-vol-94-no-47-541-560-enfr

10. "One-Dose Human Papillomavirus (HPV) Vaccine Offers Solid Protection against Cervical Cancer." (News release.) WHO, 2022.

Accessed Jan 14, 2023. www.who.int/news/item/11-04-2022-one-dose-human-papillomavirus-(hpv)-vaccine-offers-solid-protection-against-cervical-cancer

11. "Human Papillomavirus Vaccine: Supply and Demand Update." UNICEF Supply Division, 2019. www.unicef.org/supply/media/5411/file/Human-Papillomavirus-Vaccine-Market-Update-December2019.pdf

12. de Martel, C., D. Georges, F. Bray, J. Ferlay, and G. M. Clifford. "Global Burden of Cancer Attributable to Infections in 2018: A Worldwide Incidence Analysis." *Lancet Glob Health* **8**, no. 2 (Feb 2020): e180–e90. https://doi.org/10.1016/S2214-109X(19)30488-7 www.ncbi.nlm.nih.gov/pubmed/31862245

13. "HPV and Cancer." National Cancer Institute. Updated Sept 12, 2022. Accessed Jan 14, 2023. www.cancer.gov/about-cancer/causes-prevention/risk/infectious-agents/hpv-and-cancer

14. Bruni L., G. Albero, B. Serrano, *et al. Human Papillomavirus and Related Diseases in the World.* Summary report. Barcelona, Spain: ICO/ICARC HPV Information Centre, 2023. https://hpvcentre.net/statistics/reports/XWX.pdf

15. Donovan, B., N. Franklin, R. Guy, *et al.* "Quadrivalent Human Papillomavirus Vaccination and Trends in Genital Warts in Australia: Analysis of National Sentinel Surveillance Data." *Lancet Infect Dis* **11**, no. 1 (Jan 2011): 39–44. https://doi.org/10.1016/S1473-3099(10)70225-5 www.ncbi.nlm.nih.gov/pubmed/21067976

16. Drolet, M., E. Benard, N. Perez, M. Brisson, and HPV Vaccination Impact Study Group. "Population-Level Impact and Herd Effects Following the Introduction of Human Papillomavirus Vaccination Programmes: Updated Systematic Review and Meta-Analysis." *Lancet* **394**, no. 10197 (Aug 10, 2019): 497–509. https://doi.org/10.1016/S0140-6736(19)30298-3 www.ncbi.nlm.nih.gov/pubmed/31255301

17. Das, K. N. "India Develops Its First Cervical Cancer Vaccine." Reuters, 2022. Accessed Jan 14, 2023. www.reuters.com/business/healthcare-pharmaceuticals/india-develops-its-first-cervical-cancer-vaccine-2022-09-01/

18. *Prevent Protect Prosper: 2021–2025 Investment Opportunity*. Gavi: The Vaccine Alliance, 2020. www.gavi.org/sites/default/files/publications/2021-2025-Gavi-Investment-Opportunity.pdf

19. "Countries in the World by Population (2023)." Worldometer. Accessed Jan 14, 2023. www.worldometers.info/world-population /population-by-country/

20. Hollingdale, M. "New Survey Results Indicate That Nigeria Has an HIV Prevalence of 1.4%." (Press release.) UNAIDS, 2019. Accessed Jan 14, 2023. www.unaids.org/en/resources/presscentre/ pressreleaseandstatementarchive/2019/march/20190314_nigeria

21. Meites, E., P. G. Szilagyi, H. W. Chesson, *et al.* "Human Papillomavirus Vaccination for Adults: Updated Recommendations of the Advisory Committee on Immunization Practices." *MMWR Morb Mort Wkly Rep* **68**, no. 32 (Aug 16, 2019): 698–702. https://doi.org/10.15585/mmwr .mm6832a3 www.ncbi.nlm.nih.gov/pubmed/31415491

22. Olliaro, P., E. Torreele, and M. Vaillant. "COVID-19 Vaccine Efficacy and Effectiveness – the Elephant (Not) in the Room." *Lancet Microbe* **2**, no. 7 (Jul 2021): e279–e80. https://doi.org/10.1016/S2666-5247(21) 00069-0 www.ncbi.nlm.nih.gov/pubmed/33899038

Chapter 10

1. "'Finally We Can Protect Women': Japan's HPV Vaccine Battle." France 24. March 31, 2022. Accessed Jan 14, 2023. www.france24.com/en/live-news/20220331-finally-we-can-protect-women-japan-s-hpv-vaccine-battle

2. Hanley, S. J. B. "Towards the Elimination of Cervical Cancer in Japan." *J Gynecol Oncol* **32**, no. 4 (Jul 2021): e76. https://doi.org/10.3802/jgo .2021.32.e76 www.ncbi.nlm.nih.gov/pubmed/34085803

3. Mathur, P., K. Sathishkumar, M. Chaturvedi, *et al.* "Cancer Statistics, 2020: Report from National Cancer Registry Programme, India." *JCO Glob Oncol* **6** (Jul 2020): 1063–75. https://doi.org/10.1200/GO.20.00122 www.ncbi.nlm.nih.gov/pubmed/32673076

4. Bagla, P. "Indian Parliament Comes Down Hard on Cervical Cancer Trial: Panel Blasts U.S. And Indian Organizations for Alleged Ethical Lapses." *Science*, 2013. Accessed Jan 14, 2023.www.science.org/content/ article/indian-parliament-comes-down-hard-cervical-cancer-trial-rev2

5. Sankaranarayanan, R., P. Basu, P. Kaur, *et al.* "Current Status of Human Papillomavirus Vaccination in India's Cervical Cancer Prevention Efforts." *Lancet Oncol* **20**, no. 11 (Nov 2019): e637–44. https://doi.org/10.1016/S1470-2045(19)30531-5 www.ncbi.nlm.nih.gov/pubmed/31674322

6. Jones, A. "Katie Couric Feeds the HPV Vaccine 'Controversy.'" *The Atlantic*, 2013. Accessed Jan 13, 2023. www.theatlantic.com/politics/archive/2013/12/katie-couric-feeds-hpv-vaccine-controversy/355781/

7. Herper, M. "Four Ways Katie Couric Stacked the Deck against Gardasil." *Forbes*, 2013. Accessed Jan 13, 2023. www.forbes.com/sites/matthewherper/2013/12/04/four-ways-katie-couric-stacked-the-deck-against-gardasil/?sh=3a00da9a36d1

8. Holan, A. D. "Michele Bachman Says the Vaccine to Prevent HPV Can Cause Mental Retardation." *Politifact*, 2011. Accessed Jan 13, 2023. www.politifact.com/factchecks/2011/sep/16/michele-bachmann/bachmann-hpv-vaccine-cause-mental-retardation/

9. Dunn, A. G., D. Surian, J. Leask, *et al.* "Mapping Information Exposure on Social Media to Explain Differences in HPV Vaccine Coverage in the United States." *Vaccine* **35**, no. 23 (May 25, 2017): 3033–40. https://doi.org/10.1016/j.vaccine.2017.04.060 www.ncbi.nlm.nih.gov/pubmed/28461067

10. Ortiz, R. R., A. Smith, and T. Coyne-Beasley. "A Systematic Literature Review to Examine the Potential for Social Media to Impact HPV Vaccine Uptake and Awareness, Knowledge, and Attitudes About HPV and HPV Vaccination." *Hum Vaccin Immunother* **15**, no. 7–8 (2019): 1465–75. https://doi.org/10.1080/21645515.2019.1581543 www.ncbi.nlm.nih.gov/pubmed/30779682

11. Teoh, D. "The Power of Social Media for HPV Vaccination – Not Fake News!" *Am Soc Clin Oncol Educ Book* **39** (Jan 2019): 75–78. https://doi.org/10.1200/EDBK_239363 www.ncbi.nlm.nih.gov/pubmed/31099637

12. Margolis, M. A., N. T. Brewer, P. D. Shah, W. A. Calo, and M. B. Gilkey. "Stories about HPV Vaccine in Social Media, Traditional Media, and Conversations." *Prev Med* **118** (Jan 2019): 251–56. https://doi.org/10.1016/j.ypmed.2018.11.005 www.ncbi.nlm.nih.gov/pubmed/30414396

13. Mayhew, A., T. L. Mullins, L. Ding, *et al.* "Risk Perceptions and Subsequent Sexual Behaviors after HPV Vaccination in Adolescents." *Pediatrics* **133**, no. 3 (Mar 2014): 404–11. https://doi.org /10.1542/peds.2013-2822 www.ncbi.nlm.nih.gov/pubmed/24488747

14. Bednarczyk, R. A., R. Davis, K. Ault, W. Orenstein, and S. B. Omer. "Sexual Activity-Related Outcomes after Human Papillomavirus Vaccination of 11- to 12-Year-Olds." *Pediatrics* **130**, no. 5 (Nov 2012): 798–805. https://doi.org/10.1542/peds.2012-1516 www.ncbi.nlm .nih.gov/pubmed/23071201

15. Hansen, B. T. "No Evidence That HPV Vaccination Leads to Sexual Risk Compensation." *Hum Vaccin Immunother* **12**, no. 6 (Jun 2, 2016): 1451–3. https://doi.org/10.1080/21645515.2016.1158367 www .ncbi.nlm.nih.gov/pubmed/27003447

16. *Focus on the Family: 2020 Annual Report.* Focus on the Family, 2021. www.focusonthefamily.com/wp-content/uploads/2021/04/ Annual-Report-2020.pdf

17. "Focus on the Family Position Statement: HPV Vaccine." (News release.) Focus on the Family, 2019. https://media.focusonthefamily .com/topicinfo/position_statement-human_papillomavirus_vaccine .pdf

18. "Conservatives Raise Red Flag on Mandatory HPV Vaccine for Girls." *Christian Post*, 2007. www.christianpost.com/news/ conservatives-raise-red-flag-on-mandatory-hpv-vaccine-for- girls–26520/

19. "Catholic Medical Association Position Paper on HPV Immunization." (News release.) Catholic Medical Association, 2007. www.immunize.org/talking-about-vaccines/pdf/Position- Paper-on-HPV-Immunization.pdf

20. Kapp, C. "Nigerian States Again Boycott Polio-Vaccination Drive. Muslim Officials Have Rejected Assurances That the Polio Vaccine Is Safe – Leaving Africa on the Brink of Reinfection." *Lancet* **363**, no. 9410 (Feb 28, 2004): 709. https://doi.org/10.1016/s0140-6736(04) 15665-1 www.ncbi.nlm.nih.gov/pubmed/15005082

21. Ladner, J., M. H. Besson, E. Audureau, M. Rodrigues, and J. Saba. "Experiences and Lessons Learned from 29 HPV Vaccination Programs Implemented in 19 Low- and Middle-Income Countries, 2009–2014." *BMC Health Serv Res* **16**, no. 1 (Oct 13, 2016): 575.

https://doi.org/10.1186/s12913-016-1824-5 www.ncbi.nlm.nih.gov/pubmed/27737666

22. Tiley, K., E. Tessier, J. M. White, *et al.* "School-Based Vaccination Programmes: An Evaluation of School Immunisation Delivery Models in England in 2015/16." *Vaccine* **38**, no. 15 (Mar 30, 2020): 3149–56. https://doi.org/10.1016/j.vaccine.2020.01.031 www.ncbi.nlm.nih.gov/pubmed/31980192

23. Walling, E. B., N. Benzoni, J. Dornfeld, *et al.* "Interventions to Improve HPV Vaccine Uptake: A Systematic Review." *Pediatrics* **138**, no. 1 (Jul 2016): e2153863. https://doi.org/10.1542/peds.2015-3863 www.ncbi.nlm.nih.gov/pubmed/27296865

24. "HPV Vaccine: State Legislation and Regulation." National Conference of State Legislatures, 2020. Accessed Jan 13, 2023. www.ncsl.org/research/health/hpv-vaccine-state-legislation and-statutes.aspx

25. "Vaccinate before You Graduate (VBYG) Program." State of Rhode Island Department of Health. Accessed Jan 13, 2023. https://health.ri.gov/programs/detail.php?pgm_id=1010

26. Tanne, J. H. "Texas Governor Is Criticised for Decision to Vaccinate All Girls against HPV." *BMJ* **334**, no. 7589 (Feb 17, 2007): 332–3. https://doi.org/10.1136/bmj.39122.403044.DB www.ncbi.nlm.nih.gov/pubmed/17303856

27. Root, J. "Under Scrutiny, Perry Walks Back HPV Decision." *Texas Tribune*, 2011. Accessed Jan 13, 2023. www.texastribune.org/2011/08/15/facing-new-scrutiny-perry-walks-back-hpv-decision/

28. Hansen, P. R., M. Schmidtblaicher, and N. T. Brewer. "Resilience of HPV Vaccine Uptake in Denmark: Decline and Recovery." *Vaccine* **38**, no. 7 (Feb 11 2020): 1842–48. https://doi.org/10.1016/j.vaccine.2019.12.019 www.ncbi.nlm.nih.gov/pubmed/31918860

Chapter 11

1. "Smoke Alarm History." Accessed Jan 14, 2023. www.mysmokealarm.org/smoke-alarm-history/

2. Ahrens, M. "Smoke Alarms in US Home Fires." National Fire Protection Association, 2021. Accessed Jan 14, 2023. www.nfpa.org/News-and-Research/Data-research-and-tools/Detection-and-Signaling/Smoke-Alarms-in-US-Home-Fires

3. Dubner, S. J. "How Many Lives Do Smoke Alarms Really Save?" Freakonomics, 2012. https://freakonomics.com/2012/02/how-many-lives-do-smoke-alarms-really-save/

4. Chidyaonga-Maseko, F., M. L. Chirwa, and A. S. Muula. "Underutilization of Cervical Cancer Prevention Services in Low and Middle Income Countries: A Review of Contributing Factors." *Pan Afr Med J* **21** (2015): 231. https://doi.org/10.11604/pamj.2015.21.231.6350 www.ncbi.nlm.nih.gov/pubmed/26523173

5. Lott, B. E., M. J. Trejo, C. Baum, *et al.* "Interventions to Increase Uptake of Cervical Screening in Sub-Saharan Africa: A Scoping Review Using the Integrated Behavioral Model." *BMC Public Health* **20**, no. 1 (May 11, 2020): 654. https://doi.org/10.1186/s12889-020-08777-4 www.ncbi.nlm.nih.gov/pubmed/32393218

6. Gupta, R., S. Gupta, R. Mehrotra, and P. Sodhani. "Cervical Cancer Screening in Resource-Constrained Countries: Current Status and Future Directions." *Asian Pac J Cancer Prev* **18**, no. 6 (Jun 25, 2017): 1461–67. https://doi.org/10.22034/APJCP.2017.18.6.1461 www.ncbi.nlm.nih.gov/pubmed/28669152

7. Whop, L. J., G. Garvey, P. Baade, *et al.* "The First Comprehensive Report on Indigenous Australian Women's Inequalities in Cervical Screening: A Retrospective Registry Cohort Study in Queensland, Australia (2000–2011)." *Cancer* **122**, no. 10 (May 15, 2016): 1560–9. https://doi.org/10.1002/cncr.29954 www.ncbi.nlm.nih.gov/pubmed/27149550

8. "Cervical Screening in Australia: 2019." Cancer Series no. 123. Australian Institute of Health and Welfare (AIHW), 2019. Accessed Jan 14, 2023. www.aihw.gov.au/getmedia/6a9ffb2c-0c3b-45a1-b7b5-0c259bde634c/aihw-can-124.pdf.aspx?inline=true

9. *2021 Poverty Guidelines*. U.S. Department of Health and Human Services, 2021.

10. Fontham, E. T. H., A. M. D. Wolf, T. R. Church, *et al.* "Cervical Cancer Screening for Individuals at Average Risk: 2020 Guideline Update from the American Cancer Society." *CA Cancer J Clin* **70**, no. 5 (Sep 2020): 321–46. https://doi.org/10.3322/caac.21628 www.ncbi.nlm.nih.gov/pubmed/32729638

11. *WHO Guideline for Screening and Treatment of Cervical Pre-Cancer Lesions for Cervical Cancer Prevention.* 2nd ed. Geneva: World Health Organization, 2021. www.who.int/publications/i/item/9789240030824

12. Gatumo, M., S. Gacheri, A. R. Sayed, and A. Scheibe. "Women's Knowledge and Attitudes Related to Cervical Cancer and Cervical Cancer Screening in Isiolo and Tharaka Nithi Counties, Kenya: A Cross-Sectional Study." *BMC Cancer* 18, no. 1 (Jul 18, 2018): 745. https://doi.org/10.1186/s12885-018-4642-9 www.ncbi.nlm.nih.gov/pubmed/30021564

13. Perehudoff, K., H. Vermandere, A. Williams, *et al.* "Universal Cervical Cancer Control through a Right to Health Lens: Refocusing National Policy and Programmes on Underserved Women." *BMC Int Health Hum Rights* 20, no. 1 (Jul 31, 2020): 21. https://doi.org/10.1186/s12914-020-00237-9 www.ncbi.nlm.nih.gov/pubmed/32736623

14. "It Should Not Happen: Alabama's Failure to Prevent Cervical Cancer Death in the Black Belt." Human Rights Watch, 2018. Accessed Jan 14, 2023. www.hrw.org/report/2018/11/29/it-should-not-happen/alabamas-failure-prevent-cervical-cancer-death-black-belt#_ftn62

15. Freeman, L. "'We Need Access': Ending Preventable Deaths from Cervical Cancer in Rural Georgia." Human Rights Watch, 2022. www.hrw.org/report/2022/01/20/we-need-access/ending-preventable-deaths-cervical-cancer-rural-georgia

16. "Welch Allyn Kleenspec® 590 Series Premium Vaginal Specula." www.medicaldevicedepot.com/WA-KleenSpec-Vaginal-Specula-p/5900x.htm#

17. Cancer Research UK. "HPV Shame Could Put Women Off Cervical Cancer Screening." (News alert.) EurekAlert!, 2019. Accessed Jan 14, 2023. www.eurekalert.org/news-releases/582429

18. Crawford, J., F. Ahmad, D. Beaton, and A. S. Bierman. "Cancer Screening Behaviours among South Asian Immigrants in the UK, US and Canada: A Scoping Study." *Health Soc Care Community* 24, no. 2 (Mar 2016): 123–53. https://doi.org/10.1111/hsc.12208. www.ncbi.nlm.nih.gov/pubmed/25721339

19. "AICAF Infographics." Resource Types. American Indian Cancer Foundation, 2022. Accessed Jan 14, 2023. https://americanindian cancer.org/resource-types/infographics/

20. "Women Asked to 'Give Their Cervix Some Screen Time' in New Campaign." (Media release.) Manatū Hauora, Ministry of Health, 2020. Accessed Jan 14, 2023. www.health.govt.nz/news-media/ media-releases/women-asked-give-their-cervix-some-screen-time-new-campaign

21. Egiebor-Aiwan, O., I. Elhussin, D. Nganwa, *et al.* "The Impact of Race and Geographical Location on the Treatment Options of Cervical Cancer in Black and White Women Living in the State of Alabama." *J Healthc Sci Humanit* **10**, no. 1 (Fall 2020): 40–60. www.ncbi.nlm.nih .gov/pubmed/35106184

22. Ford, S., W. Tarraf, K. P. Williams, L. A. Roman, and R. Leach. "Differences in Cervical Cancer Screening and Follow-Up for Black and White Women in the United States." *Gynecol Oncol* **160**, no. 2 (Feb 2021): 369–74.

23. Johnson, M., C. Wakefield, and K. Garthe. "Qualitative Socioecological Factors of Cervical Cancer Screening Use among Transgender Men." *Prev Med Rep* **17** (Mar 2020): 101052. https://doi .org/10.1016/j.pmedr.2020.101052 www.ncbi.nlm.nih.gov /pubmed/32021762

24. Dhillon, N., J. L. Oliffe, M. T. Kelly, and J. Krist. "Bridging Barriers to Cervical Cancer Screening in Transgender Men: A Scoping Review." *Am J Mens Health* **14**, no. 3 (May-Jun 2020): 1557988320925691. https://doi.org/10.1177/1557988320925691 www.ncbi.nlm.nih.gov/pubmed/32489142

25. Fischer, F., K. Lange, K. Klose, W. Greiner, and A. Kraemer. "Barriers and Strategies in Guideline Implementation – A Scoping Review." *Healthcare (Basel)* **4**, no. 3 (Jun 29, 2016): 36. https://doi.org/ 10.3390/healthcare4030036 www.ncbi.nlm.nih.gov/pubmed/ 27417624

26. *Improving Public Investments in the Health Sector in the Context of COVID-19.* Health Budget Brief. UNICEF Malawi Health, 2021. www .unicef.org/esa/media/8991/file/UNICEF-Malawi-2020-2021-Health-Budget-Brief.pdf

27. Gossa, W., and M. D. Fetters. "How Should Cervical Cancer Prevention Be Improved in LMICs?" *AMA J Ethics* **22**, no. 2 (Feb 1, 2020): E126–34. https://doi.org/10.1001/amajethics.2020.126 www .ncbi.nlm.nih.gov/pubmed/32048583

28. Boom, K., M. Lopez, M. Daheri, *et al.* "Perspectives on Cervical Cancer Screening and Prevention: Challenges Faced by Providers and Patients along the Texas–Mexico Border." *Perspect Public Health* **139**, no. 4 (Jul 2019): 199–205. https://doi.org/10.1177/ 1757913918793443 https://pubmed.ncbi.nlm.nih.gov/30117782/

29. "Women's Health Insurance Coverage." Women's Health Policy, KFF, 2022. Accessed Jan 14, 2023. www.kff.org/womens-health-policy/fact-sheet/womens-health-insurance-coverage/#

30. *Eligibility Overview: Washington Apple Health (Medicaid) Programs.* Washington State Health Care Authority, 2022. www.hca.wa.gov/ assets/free-or-low-cost/22-315.pdf

31. Sabik, L. M., W. W. Tarazi, and C. J. Bradley. "State Medicaid Expansion Decisions and Disparities in Women's Cancer Screening." *Am J Prev Med* **48**, no. 1 (Jan 2015): 98–103. https://doi .org/10.1016/j.amepre.2014.08.015 www.ncbi.nlm.nih.gov/ pubmed/25441234

32. "Cancer Statistics Center: Cancer Type: Cervix." American Cancer Society, 2022. Accessed Jan 14, 2023. https://cancerstatisticscenter .cancer.org/#!/cancer-site/Cervix

33. Francoeur, A. A., C.-I. Liao, M. A. Caesar, *et al.* "The Increasing Incidence of Stage IV Cervical Cancer in the USA: What Factors Are Related?" *Int J Gynecol Cancer* (Aug 18, 2022). https://doi.org/10.1136/ ijgc-2022-003728 www.ncbi.nlm.nih.gov/pubmed/35981903

34. *Planned Parenthood: 2019–2020 Annual Report.* Planned Parenthood, 2020. www.plannedparenthood.org/uploads/filer_public/67/30/ 67305ea1-8da2-4cee-9191-19228c1d6f70/210219-annual-report-2019-2020-web-final.pdf

35. "This Is Who We Are: Creating a Healthier World for Women, Men, and Young People." (Fact sheet.) Planned Parenthood, 2021. Accessed Jan 10, 2023. www.plannedparenthood.org/uploads/ filer_public/2d/e1/2de1e14c-9bce-46b8-94f5-d57de80f1a3d/210210-fact-sheet-who-we-are-p01.pdf

Chapter 12

1. *Global Strategy to Accelerate the Elimination of Cervical Cancer as a Public Health Problem.* World Health Organization, 2020. www.who.int/pub lications/i/item/9789240014107

2. Burundi, Central African Republic, Chad, Rwanda, Sierra Leone, South Sudan, Togo, and Afghanistan are all countries without an oncologist. Mathew, A. "Global Survey of Clinical Oncology Workforce." *J Glob Oncol* **4** (Sep 2018): 1–12. https://doi.org/10.1200/ JGO.17.00188 www.ncbi.nlm.nih.gov/pubmed/30241241

3. "Total Population of Canada from 2017 to 2027." Statista, 2022. Accessed Jan 13, 2023. www.statista.com/statistics/263742/ total-population-in-canada/

4. Zubizarreta, E., and E. Rosenblatt, eds. *Radiotherapy in Cancer Care: Facing the Global Challenge.* Austria: International Atomic Energy Agency, 2017. www-pub.iaea.org/MTCD/Publications/PDF/ P1638_web.pdf

5. Duska, L. R. "Access to Quality Gynecologic Oncology Care: A Work in Progress." *Cancer* **124**, no. 13 (Jul 1, 2018): 2680–83. https://doi.org/ 10.1002/cncr.31391 www.ncbi.nlm.nih.gov/pubmed/29767847

6. Minig, L., P. Padilla-Iserte, and C. Zorrero. "The Relevance of Gynecologic Oncologists to Provide High-Quality of Care to Women with Gynecological Cancer." *Front Oncol* **5** (2015): 308. https://doi.org/ 10.3389/fonc.2015.00308 www.ncbi.nlm.nih.gov/pubmed/ 26835417

7. *National Framework for Gynaecological Cancer Control Appendix C,* Table C-1. Surry Hills, NSW: Cancer Australia, 2016.

8. Barrington, D. A., S. E. Dilley, E. E. Landers, *et al.* "Distance from a Comprehensive Cancer Center: A Proxy for Poor Cervical Cancer Outcomes?" *Gynecologic Oncology* **143**, no. 3 (2016): 617–21. https://doi.org /10.1016/j.ygyno.2016.10.004

9. Temkin, S. M., S. A. Fleming, S. Amrane, N. Schluterman, and M. Terplan. "Geographic Disparities amongst Patients with Gynecologic Malignancies at an Urban NCI-Designated Cancer Center." *Gynecologic Oncology* **137**, no. 3 (2015): 497–502. https://doi .org/10.1016/j.ygyno.2015.03.010

10. van Schalkwyk, S. L., J. E. Maree, and S. C. Wright. "Cervical Cancer: The Route from Signs and Symptoms to Treatment in South Africa." *Reprod Health Matters* **16**, no. 32 (Nov 2008): 9–17. https://doi.org/10.1016/S0968-8080(08)32399-4 www.ncbi.nlm.nih.gov/pubmed/19027618

11. Moodley, J., F. M. Walter, S. E. Scott, and A. M. Mwaka. "Towards Timely Diagnosis of Symptomatic Breast and Cervical Cancer in South Africa." *S Afr Med J* **108**, no. 10 (Oct 2, 2018): 803–4. https://doi.org/10.7196/SAMJ.2018.v108i10.13478 www.ncbi.nlm.nih.gov/pubmed/30421705

12. Egiebor-Aiwan, O., I. Elhussin, D. Nganwa, *et al.* "The Impact of Race and Geographical Location on the Treatment Options of Cervical Cancer in Black and White Women Living in the State of Alabama." *J Healthc Sci Humanit* **10**, no. 1 (Fall 2020): 40–60. www.ncbi.nlm.nih.gov/pubmed/35106184

13. Fleming, S., N. H. Schluterman, J. K. Tracy, and S. M. Temkin. "Black and White Women in Maryland Receive Different Treatment for Cervical Cancer." *PLOS ONE* **9**, no. 8 (2014): e104344. https://doi.org/10.1371/journal.pone.0104344 www.ncbi.nlm.nih.gov/pubmed/25121587

14. Kotha, N. V., C. W. Williamson, L. K. Mell, *et al.* "Disparities in Time to Start of Definitive Radiation Treatment for Patients with Locally Advanced Cervical Cancer." *Int J Gynecol Cancer* **32**, no. 5 (May 3, 2022): 613–18. https://doi.org/10.1136/ijgc-2021-003305 www.ncbi.nlm.nih.gov/pubmed/35428688

Chapter 13

1. Benoit, M. F., J. F. Ma, and B. A. Upperman. "Comparison of 2015 Medicare Relative Value Units for Gender-Specific Procedures: Gynecologic and Gynecologic-Oncologic versus Urologic CPT Coding. Has Time Healed Gender-Worth?" *Gynecol Oncol* **144**, no. 2 (2017): 336–42. https://doi.org/10.1016/j.ygyno.2016.12.006

2. Cherouny, P., and C. Nadolski. "Underreimbursement of Obstetric and Gynecologic Invasive Services by the Resource-Based Relative Value Scale." *Obstet Gynecol* **87**, no. 3

(Mar 1996): 328–31. https://doi.org/10.1016/0029-7844(95)00442-4 www.ncbi.nlm.nih.gov/pubmed/8598949

3. Polan, R. M., and E. L. Barber. "Reimbursement for Female-Specific Compared with Male-Specific Procedures over Time." *Obstet Gynecol* **138**, no. 6 (Dec 1, 2021): 878–83. https://doi.org/10.1097/AOG .0000000000004599 www.ncbi.nlm.nih.gov/pubmed/34736273

4. Kane, L. "Physician Compensation Report: Incomes Gain, Pay Gaps Remain." *Medscape*, 2022. www.medscape.com/slideshow/ 2022-compensation-overview-6015043?faf=1#32

5. Dossa, F., A. N. Simpson, R. Sutradhar, *et al.* "Sex-Based Disparities in the Hourly Earnings of Surgeons in the Fee-for-Service System in Ontario, Canada." *JAMA Surg* **154**, no. 12 (Dec 1, 2019): 1134–42. https://doi.org/10.1001/jamasurg.2019.3769 www.ncbi.nlm.nih.gov/ pubmed/31577348

6. "UICC Members Regional Meeting – Latin America and the Caribbean." World Cancer Congress, 2018. www.worldcancercongress.org/sites/congress/files/atoms/files/ Regional%20meeting.pdf

7. "Breaking the Silos: Empowering Adolescent Girls and Young Women to Access Integrated Health-Care Services." (News release.) UNAIDS, 2016. www.unaids.org/sites/default/files/ 20160608_PR_HLM_OAFLA_rev.pdf

8. Karanja-Chege, C. M. "HPV Vaccination in Kenya: The Challenges Faced and Strategies to Increase Uptake." *Front Public Health* **10** (2022): 802947. https://doi.org/10.3389/fpubh.2022.802947 www.ncbi.nlm.nih.gov/pubmed/35387182

9. Habib, J. "Women Are Championing HPV Vaccine Campaigns in Kenya." *Global Citizen*, 2020. Accessed Jan 15, 2023. www.globalcitizen .org/de/content/women-championing-hpv-vaccine-kenya/

10. Low, N., M. F. Chersich, K. Schmidlin, *et al.* "Intravaginal Practices, Bacterial Vaginosis, and HIV Infection in Women: Individual Participant Data Meta-Analysis." *PLoS Med* **8**, no. 2 (Feb 15, 2011): e1000416. https://doi.org/10.1371/journal.pmed.1000416 www .ncbi.nlm.nih.gov/pubmed/21358808

11. McClelland, R. S., L. Lavreys, W. M. Hassan, *et al.* "Vaginal Washing and Increased Risk of HIV-1 Acquisition among African Women: A 10-Year Prospective Study." *AIDS* **20**, no. 2 (Jan 9, 2006): 269–73.

https://doi.org/10.1097/01.aids.0000196165.48518.7b www.ncbi
.nlm.nih.gov/pubmed/16511421

12. Ferrant, G. "Unpaid Care Work: The Missing Link in the Analysis of
Gender Gaps in Labour Outcomes." OECD Development Centre,
2014. www.oecd.org/dev/development-gender/Unpaid_care_work
.pdf

13. Organisation for Economic Co-operation and Development. *Sigi
2021 Regional Report for Africa.* Paris: OECD Publishing, 2021.
https://doi.org/10.1787/a6d95d90-en

14. Clare C., P. E. Revollo, R. Harvey Max, *et al. Time to Care: Unpaid and
Underpaid Care Work and the Global Inequality Crisis.* Cowley: Oxfam
International, 2020. https://oxfamilibrary.openrepository.com/
bitstream/handle/10546/620928/bp-time-to-care-inequality-
200120 en.pdf

15. Seedat, S., and M. Rondon. "Women's Wellbeing and the Burden of
Unpaid Work." *BMJ* **374** (Aug 31, 2021): n1972. https://doi.org/10
.1136/bmj.n1972 www.ncbi.nlm.nih.gov/pubmed/34465574

16. "Providing Unpaid Household and Care Work in the United States:
Uncovering Inequality." Economic, Security, Mobility, and Equity,
Institute for Women's Policy Research, 2020. Accessed Jan 15,
2023. https://iwpr.org/iwpr-issues/esme/providing-unpaid-
household-and-care-work-in-the-united-states-uncovering-
inequality/

17. Samtleben, C. "Care and Careers: Gender (in)Equality in Unpaid
Care, Housework and Employment." *Res Soc Stratif Mobil* **77** (2020):
100659.

18. Cook, E. E., A. S. Venkataramani, J. J. Kim, R. M. Tamimi, and
M. D. Holmes. "Legislation to Increase Uptake of HPV Vaccination
and Adolescent Sexual Behaviors." *Pediatrics* **142**, no. 3 (Sep 2018):
e20180458. https://doi.org/10.1542/peds.2018-0458 www.ncbi.nlm
.nih.gov/pubmed/30104422

19. Brouwer, A. F., R. L. Delinger, M. C. Eisenberg, *et al.* "HPV
Vaccination Has Not Increased Sexual Activity or Accelerated
Sexual Debut in a College-Aged Cohort of Men and Women." *BMC
Public Health* **19**, no. 1 (Jun 25, 2019): 821. https://doi.org/10.1186/
s12889-019-7134-1 www.ncbi.nlm.nih.gov/pubmed/31238911

20. Jena, A. B., D. P. Goldman, and S. A. Seabury. "Incidence of Sexually Transmitted Infections after Human Papillomavirus Vaccination among Adolescent Females." *JAMA Intern Med* **175**, no. 4 (Apr 2015): 617–23. https://doi.org/10.1001/jamainternmed.2014.7886 www.ncbi.nlm.nih.gov/pubmed/25664968

21. Turiho, A. K., W. W. Muhwezi, E. S. Okello, *et al.* "Human Papillomavirus (HPV) Vaccination and Adolescent Girls' Knowledge and Sexuality in Western Uganda: A Comparative Cross-Sectional Study." *PLoS One* **10**, no. 9 (2015): e0137094. https://doi.org/10.1371/journal.pone.0137094 www.ncbi.nlm.nih.gov/pubmed/26327322

22. Frio, G. S., and M. T. A. Franca. "Human Papillomavirus Vaccine and Risky Sexual Behavior: Regression Discontinuity Design Evidence from Brazil." *Econ Hum Biol* **40** (Jan 2021): 100946. https://doi.org/ 10.1016/j.ehb.2020.100946 www.ncbi.nlm.nih.gov/pubmed/33264703

23. "Facts About HPV and the HPV Vaccine." Cancer Council Victoria. Accessed Jan 14, 2023. www.hpvvaccine.org.au/parents/myths-and-facts-about-hpv-and-the-vaccine.aspx

24. Alcala, H. E., E. Mitchell, and J. Keim-Malpass. "Adverse Childhood Experiences and Cervical Cancer Screening." *J Womens Health (Larchmt)* **26**, no. 1 (Jan 2017): 58–63. https://doi.org/10.1089/ jwh.2016.5823 www.ncbi.nlm.nih.gov/pubmed/27500413

25. "Victims of Sexual Violence: Statistics." RAINN. Accessed Jan 22, 2023. www.rainn.org/statistics/victims-sexual-violence

Chapter 14

1. White, H. "Opinion: Zambia – Leading the Way toward Ending Cervical Cancer." *Devex*, 2022. www.devex.com/news/sponsored/opinion-zambia-leading-the-way-toward-ending-cervical-cancer-104303

2. "How Rwanda Is Improving Uptake of HPV Immunisation." apolitical, 2020. Accessed Jan 14, 2023. https://apolitical.co/solution-articles/en/how-rwanda-is-improving-uptake-of-hpv-immunisation

3. Barnabas, R. V., E. R. Brown, M. A. Onono, *et al.* "Efficacy of Single-Dose HPV Vaccination among Young African Women." *NEJM Evid* **1**, no. 5 (Jun 2022): EVIDoa2100056. https://doi.org/10.1056/ EVIDoa2100056 www.ncbi.nlm.nih.gov/pubmed/35693874

4. *WHO HPV Vaccine Global Market Study, April 2022.* WHO, 2022. Accessed Jan 14, 2023. www.who.int/publications/m/item/who-hpv-vaccine-global-market-study-april–2022

5. "Cecolin®." Vaccines, 2022. (WHO – Prequalification of Medical Products [IVDs, Medicines, Vaccines and Immunization Devices, Vector Control]). https://extranet.who.int/pqweb/content/cecolin®

6. "HPV Associated Disorders Global Market Report 2022: Ukraine-Russia War Impact." Reportlinker, 2022. Accessed Jan 15, 2023. www.globenewswire.com/news-release/2022/12/20/2576899/0/en/HPV-Associated-Disorders-Global-Market-Report-2022-Ukraine-Russia-War-Impact.html#

7. Lemay, A., K. Hoebel, C. P. Bridge, *et al.* "Improving the Repeatability of Deep Learning Models with Monte Carlo Dropout." *NPJ Digit Med* **5**, no. 1 (Nov 18, 2022): 174. https://doi.org/10.1038/s41746-022-00709-3 www.ncbi.nlm.nih.gov/pubmed/36400939

8. Desai, K. T., B. Befano, Z. Xue, *et al.* "The Development of 'Automated Visual Evaluation' for Cervical Cancer Screening: The Promise and Challenges in Adapting Deep-Learning for Clinical Testing: Interdisciplinary Principles of Automated Visual Evaluation in Cervical Screening." *Int J Cancer* **150**, no. 5 (Mar 1, 2022): 741–52. https://doi.org/10.1002/ijc.33879 www.ncbi.nlm.nih.gov/pubmed/34800038

9. PEPFAR countries include Botswana, Eswatini, Ethiopia, Kenya, Lesotho, Malawi, Mozambique, Namibia, Tanzania, Uganda, Zambia, Zimbabwe. "Go Further Country Fact Sheets: The United States President's Emergency Plan for Aids Relief." U.S. Department of State, updated July 9, 2020. Accessed Jan 14, 2023. www.state.gov/go-further-country-fact-sheets/

10. Godfrey, C., A. Prainito, I. Lapidos-Salaiz, M. Barnhart, and D. H. Watts. "Reducing Cervical Cancer Deaths in Women Living with HIV: PEPFAR and the Go Further Partnership." *Prev Med* **144** (Mar 2021): 106295. https://doi.org/10.1016/j.ypmed.2020.106295 www.ncbi.nlm.nih.gov/pubmed/33678226

11. Winer, R. L., A. A. Gonzales, C. J. Noonan, and D. S. Buchwald. "A Cluster-Randomized Trial to Evaluate a Mother-Daughter Dyadic Educational Intervention for Increasing HPV Vaccination Coverage in American Indian Girls." *J Community Health* **41**, no. 2 (Apr 2016):

274–81. https://doi.org/10.1007/s10900-015-0093-2 www.ncbi .nlm.nih.gov/pubmed/26399648

12. "Join AICAF on January 20, 2022 to Celebrate Turquoise Thursday!" Turquoise Thursday, Cervical Cancer Awareness Month 2022. American Indian Cancer Foundation. Accessed Jan 14, 2023. https://americanindiancancer.org/aicaf-project/turquoise/

13. "AICAF Infographics." Resource Types. American Indian Cancer Foundation, 2022. Accessed Jan 14, 2023. https:// americanindian cancer.org/resource-types/infographics/

14. Lott, B. E., B. O. Okusanya, E. J. Anderson, *et al.* "Interventions to Increase Uptake of Human Papillomavirus (HPV) Vaccination in Minority Populations: A Systematic Review." *Prev Med Rep* **19** (Sep 2020): 101163. https://doi.org/10.1016/j.pmedr.2020.101163 www.ncbi.nlm.nih.gov/pubmed/32714778

15. Christensen, A. "Navajo Nation Home to Region's Highest HPV Vaccination Rate." University of Arizona, Cancer Center, 2018. Accessed Jan 22, 2023. https://cancercenter.arizona.edu/news/2018/ 04/navajo-nation-home-region's-highest-hpv-vaccination-rate

16. "General Health: Cervical Cancer Screening." LGBT Foundation. Accessed September 17, 2020. https://lgbt.foundation/screening

17. "Improving Cancer Care for the LGBTQ+ Community." *Cancer News*, Cancer Research UK, 2021. Accessed Jan 15, 2023. https://news .cancerresearchuk.org/2021/07/26/improving-cancer-care-for-the-lgbtq-community/

18. "Canada Acts to Meet WHO Call to Eliminate Cervical Cancer." Canadian Partnership Against Cancer, 2020. Accessed Jan 22, 2023. www.partnershipagainstcancer.ca/news-events/news/article/ eliminate-cervical-cancer/

19. Ahmed, S., R. K. Shahid, and J. A. Episkenew. "Disparity in Cancer Prevention and Screening in Aboriginal Populations: Recommendations for Action." *Curr Oncol* **22**, no. 6 (Dec 2015): 417–26. https://doi.org/10.3747/co.22.2599 www.ncbi.nlm.nih.gov/ pubmed/26715875

20. "Women Asked to 'Give Their Cervix Some Screen Time' in New Campaign." (Media release.) Manatū Hauora, Ministry of Health, 2020. Accessed Jan 15, 2023. www.health.govt.nz/news-media/

media-releases/women-asked-give-their-cervix-some-screen-time-new-campaign

21. "Cancers Caused by HPV Are Preventable." Centers for Disease Control and Prevention, updated Nov 1, 2021. Accessed Jan 15, 2023. www.cdc.gov/hpv/hcp/protecting-patients.html

22. Pingali, C., D. Yankey, L. D. Elam-Evans, *et al.* "National Vaccination Coverage among Adolescents Aged 13–17 Years – National Immunization Survey-Teen, United States, 2021." *MMWR Morb Mortal Wkly Rep* **71**, no. 35 (Sep 2, 2022): 1101–08. https://doi.org/10.15585/mmwr.mm7135a1 www.ncbi.nlm.nih.gov/pubmed/36048724

23. Hall, M. T., K. T. Simms, J. B. Lew, *et al.* "Projected Future Impact of HPV Vaccination and Primary HPV Screening on Cervical Cancer Rates from 2017–2035: Example from Australia." *PLoS One* **13**, no. 2 (2018): e0185332. https://doi.org/10.1371/journal.pone.0185332 www.ncbi.nlm.nih.gov/pubmed/29444073

24. "Cervical Cancer: This Daffodil Day, You're Giving to Cervical Cancer Research." Cancer Council Daffodil Day Appeal. Accessed Jan 15, 2023. www.daffodilday.com.au/your-impact/research/cervical-cancer.

25. Canfell, K. "Australia On-Track to Be the First Country to Achieve Cervical Cancer Elimination." HPV World. Accessed Jan 15, 2023. www.hpvworld.com/articles/australia-on-track-to-be-the-first-country-to-achieve-cervical-cancer-elimination/

26. Farnsworth, A. "Cervical Cancer Screening in Australia: Past, Present and Future." *Common Sense Pathology* (2015): 1–8. www.rcpa.edu.au/getattachment/7c4c60ca-35fd-4338-bf80-392e25dd200a/Cervical-Cancer-Screening-in-Australia.aspx

27. Donovan, B., N. Franklin, R. Guy, *et al.* "Quadrivalent Human Papillomavirus Vaccination and Trends in Genital Warts in Australia: Analysis of National Sentinel Surveillance Data." *Lancet Infect Dis* **11**, no. 1 (Jan 2011): 39–44. https://doi.org/10.1016/S1473-3099(10)70225-5 www.ncbi.nlm.nih.gov/pubmed/21067976

28. "NSW Cancer Plan: 2016–2021. Focus: Aboriginal Communities." Cancer Institute NSW. www.cancer.nsw.gov.au/about-cancer/document-library/nsw-cancer-plan-2016-2021/focus-aboriginal-communities

29. *Global Strategy to Accelerate the Elimination of Cervical Cancer as a Public Health Problem.* Geneva: World Health Organization, 2020. www.who.int/publications/i/item/9789240014107

30. "World Health Assembly Adopts Global Strategy to Accelerate Cervical Cancer Elimination." World Health Organization, 2020. www.who.int/news/item/19-08-2020-world-health-assembly-adopts-global-strategy-to-accelerate-cervical-cancer-elimination

Chapter 15

1. Hall, M. T., M. A. Smith, K. T. Simms, *et al.* "The Past, Present and Future Impact of HIV Prevention and Control on HPV and Cervical Disease in Tanzania: A Modelling Study." *PLoS One* **15**, no. 5 (2020): e0231388. https://doi.org/10.1371/journal.pone.0231388 www.ncbi.nlm.nih.gov/pubmed/32374729

2. Grund, J. M., T. S. Bryant, I. Jackson, *et al.* "Association between Male Circumcision and Women's Biomedical Health Outcomes: A Systematic Review." *Lancet Glob Health* **5**, no. 11 (Nov 2017): e1113-22. https://doi.org/10.1016/S2214-109X(17)30369-8 www.ncbi.nlm.nih.gov/pubmed/29025633

3. Centers for Disease Control and Prevention. "Recommendations on the Use of Quadrivalent Human Papillomavirus Vaccine in Males – Advisory Committee on Immunization Practices (ACIP), 2011." *MMWR Morb Mortal Wkly Rep* **60**, no. 50 (Dec 23, 2011): 1705–08. www.ncbi.nlm.nih.gov/pubmed/22189893

4. "Meeting of the Strategic Advisory Group of Experts on Immunization, October 2019: Conclusions and Recommendations." *Wkly Epidemiol Rec* **94**, no. 47 (Nov 22, 2019): 541–60. https://reliefweb.int/report/world/weekly-epidemiological-record-wer-22-november-2019-vol-94-no-47-541-560-enfr

5. Bruni, L., A. Saura-Lazaro, A. Montoliu, *et al.* "HPV Vaccination Introduction Worldwide and WHO and UNICEF Estimates of National HPV Immunization Coverage 2010–2019." *Prev Med* **144** (Mar 2021): 106399. https://doi.org/10.1016/j.ypmed.2020.106399 www.ncbi.nlm.nih.gov/pubmed/33388322

INDEX